OSTEOARTHRITIS RHEUMATISMS ARTHRITIS

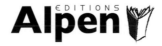

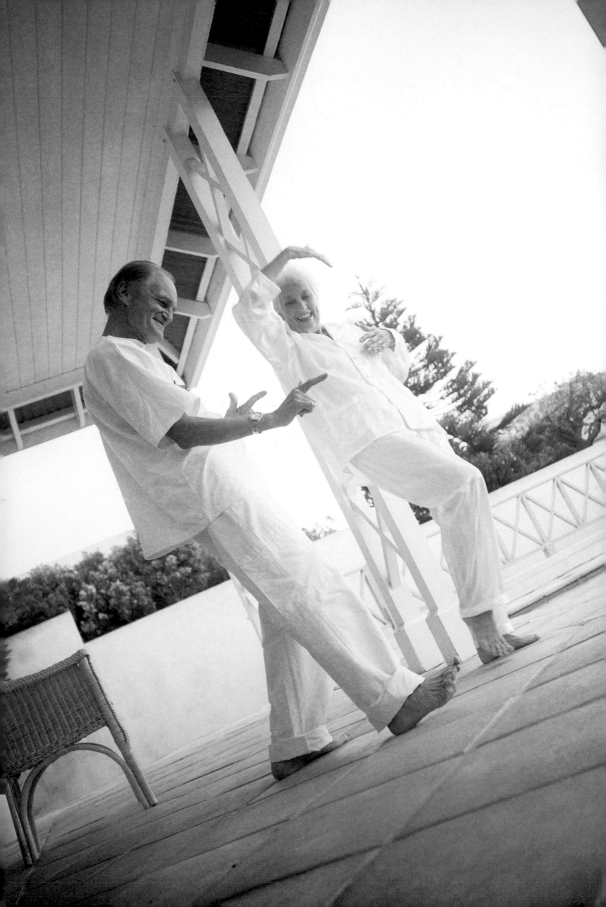

Doctors Charlotte Tourmente and Max Tétau

OSTEOARTHRITIS RHEUMATISMS ARTHRITIS

Natural solutions which will change your life

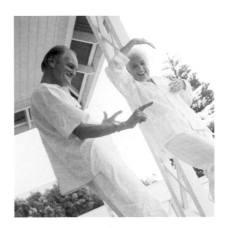

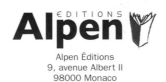

Alpen Éditions
9, avenue Albert II
98000 Monaco

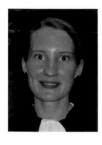

Charlotte Tourmente general medicine intern at the Nancy School of Medicine.
She is also a medical journalist and would like to devote herself to writing medical books for the general public.

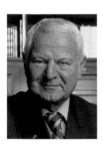

Dr. Max Tétau has practiced homeopathy and phytotherapy for many years. He is the editor in chief of Cahiers de Biothérapie and author of numerous works primarily dedicated to the use of plants in medicine. He is the chairman of the Biotherapy Medical Society, National and International Homeopathy Federations and International Phytotherapy Federation. Due to the numerous scientific works her has dedicated to these disciplines he is considered an authority in the world for alternative medicine.

Exclusive copyrights:
© Alpen Éditions
9, avenue Albert II
MC - 98000 MONACO
Tel: 00377 97 77 62 10
Fax: 00377 97 77 62 11
Web: www.alpen.mc

Managing Publisher: Christophe Didierlaurent
Editorial: Fabienne Desmarets and Sandra Del Barba
Designer: Stéphane Falaschi

Copyrights:
Brand X Pictures, Digital Vision, Eye Wire, Image Source, Photo Alto, Photo Disc, Scorpius

Artwork: © Sébastien Telleschi

ISBN13: 978-2-35934-065-5
Printed in Italy

Introduction

Osteoarthritis....Your grandmother complains of it often, your neighbor has it, or maybe even you do. And even if it hasn't started yet, don't you feel you joints getting weaker as the years pass?

Osteoarthritis is the most common joint disorder. It afflicts 17% of the population. If older people suffer the most, they are not the only ones to do so. But the terms osteoarthritis is often used "wildly": people mix up rheumatisms, polyarthritis or even gout very easily. Nothing is more normal! They all have different origins but all affect the joints. So what is osteoarthritis?

How does it appear? What are the disorders it can be mixed up with? Once a diagnosis is clearly established, how is it treated? What drugs are taken, is surgery necessary and why can't plant remedies be used? Some are of formidable effectiveness for relieving joint pain.

Many of these questions will be addressed in this book which will also help you discover that diet plays a role as well. Even if treated, osteoarthritis can

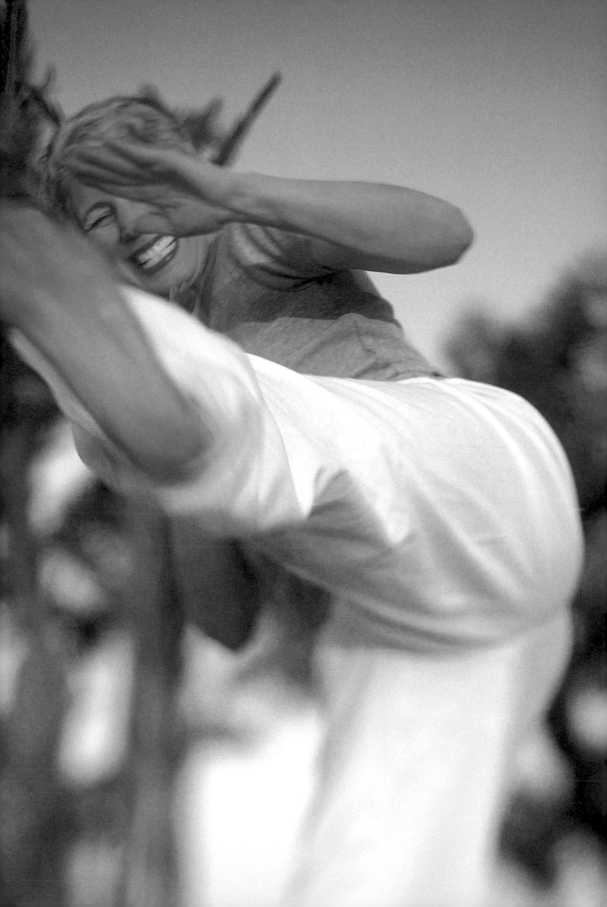

cause problems in daily life. Practicing a sport can be really beneficial. So move yes, but not just any which way! Did you know that some everyday movements can actually worsen the disease? It is important to avoid them and re-establish correct movements. In the end of the book you'll find a description of good positions to use in daily life to protect your joints and live comfortably with your osteoarthritis.

Even if not necessarily exhaustive, the main aim of this book is to answer the questions you ask yourself. It also wants to improve your daily life or that of people around you who are affected or suffering.

If this is the case when you close the book we will have reached our goal.

TABLE OF CONTENTS

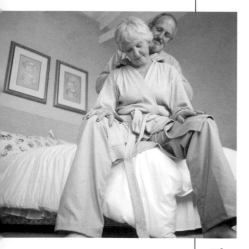

OSTEOARTHRITIS, WHAT IS IT?

When joints show signs of fatigue

Pain is the first symptom of osteoarthritis...when it occurs the process has already begun. In some individuals, osteoarthritis may even remain completely silent!

The pain varies, at times faint and mild and sometimes very strong. Normally at the beginning, it appears after exertion, like a long walk, but it is still bearable. It disappears with rest. Then, as time goes on, the osteoarthritis progresses, the pain gets stronger and occurs with even the slightest movement. Over the years, the joint becomes painful, even when resting and during the night.

"I feel stiff."

When you wake up, you feel like your body can't move! In the beginning, the stiffness doesn't last very long: it ends quickly. It's as if you were completely "out of shape" or very numb: for example, you have a hard time bending your knee to get up and you often have to wait to recover some of your flexibility. This is what is called "morning loosening up ». Based on the individual and the disease's progression, this can last for a few minutes to a few hours. This feeling of not being able to normally use your limbs also occurs throughout the day. Joints have a tendency to lock when you stay still for too long to see a movie or during a ride in the car. There is also "mechanical" pain, the joint seizes up, it no longer works normally..

Sleep and pain

Many people who suffer from osteoarthritis complain of nighttime pain (up to 60% according to studies). This pain disturbs sleep, but it also seems that in return the lack of sleep exacerbates the sensation of pain. It is important to talk about this with your doctor, to describe your symptoms precisely so that he or she can treat this aspect of the disease..

"I creak like the floor!"

You often hear about creaking joints, doctors call it "crepitus", which appears when the osteoarthritis has already evolved substantially. The famous "creak" is heard more during movement of the knee, rarely of the hip. It often affects the fingers. The intensity of the noise can be surprising, but normally this loud noise doesn't hurt! The patient feels a slightly strange "faint" sensation. The noise simply comes from a bone sliding against the other bone in the joint when the cartilage is no longer there to soften the movement.

Each age has its own osteoarthritis

The osteoarthritis that causes many to suffer after age 45 is a slow and almost "normal" evolution: it is simply due to aging of the skeleton. It essentially strikes the hips and knees, the two joints which support the body. The fingers, lumbar (lower back) and cervical (in the neck) vertebrae may also be affected. When osteoarthritis occurs before age 40, it is most often the consequence of a problem occurring in the joint: it may be due to a joint infection, loose ligaments, a trauma or injury, a metabolic imbalance (for example gout) or even following an operation on a joint.

Where does osteoarthritis start?

Osteoarthritis first acts on the joints which support the body. Then it affects the knee, on just one side. The other knee will be reached later, or less significantly. The hips are the second most frequent site affected by osteoarthritis. Afterwards, it is often the upper or lower back vertebrae or the fingers which suffer.

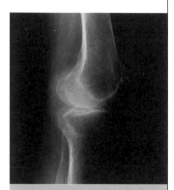

Cartilage

This is a bluish white, smooth substance that resembles rubber. Elastic, very supple and also resistant, it is composed of cells called chondrocytes, which allow it to renew itself, collagen fibers and large spongy molecules. There are four types of cartilage:
- synchondrosis epiphyseos which permits bone growth in children;
- the very soft auricular cartilage;
- a very fibrous cartilage in the knee semilunar cartilage;
- hyaline cartilage which covers the ends of the bones, at the joints. This is the one which is damaged by osteoarthritis.

When joints simply wear out

Osteoarthritis is a chronic rheumatism which afflicts 17% of population. It is closely tied to age: after age 65, one person out of two suffers from it. Osteoarthritis is due to the progressive destruction of joint cartilage. When the cartilage loses the suppleness and elasticity that lets it ensure proper operation of the joints, the mechanism seizes up. The thickness of the cartilage which covers the end of the bones at the joints decreases and no longer softens the friction between bones.

To illustrate the case of osteoarthritis, you can look at an affected knee as an example (*see the diagram*). But the same is true for all very mobile joints, such as those of the hips or fingers. In all these cases, when the cartilage is eroded by osteoarthritis, it can no longer manage to protect the joints.

Progressive cartilage erosion

Cartilage erosion starts well before the first pain occurs. On top of eroding, the cartilage wears out, it fissures, becomes weaker and cracks; the afflicted joint becomes more and more painful. The bone is progressively damaged by the friction it directly undergoes. The body has protective means: chondrocytes, or builder cells, try to produce cartilage in order to compensate for what is lost. But, unfortunately this is often not enough and the cartilage continues to erode. Attempts to repair then

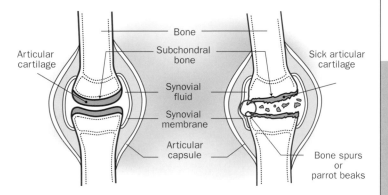

Bone
Subchondral bone
Articular cartilage
Synovial fluid
Synovial membrane
Articular capsule
Sick articular cartilage
Bone spurs or parrot beaks

Diagram of a healthy joint and a diseased joint.

In the diagram cartilage is present on the bone on both sides of the joint. In the center a capsule connects the two bones. It is covered with a membrane which secrets synovial fluid, a lubricant for the joint. The cartilage's role is to absorb the synovial fluid when the knee is at rest and return this liquid when walking, in order to play a protective role. The pressure of the body on the knee and the movement compress the cartilage which is "squeezed" like a sponge and then sends the synovial fluid to the joint. This coming and going of fluid during movements allows walking to progress correctly and all the effort of the knee. When the cartilage is eroded by osteoarthritis, it no longer manages to correctly distribute the synovial fluid and to protect the joints.

result in small bony growths which deform the joint: these are the famous "parrot beaks" or osteophytes, which are also called bone spurs. This is the stage when inflammation normally appears. In the most severe cases, the cartilage totally disappears.

Osteoarthritis, an inflammatory disease

Inflammation is a reaction mechanism of tissues when they perceive a threat. It was long believed that osteoarthritis was not an inflammatory disease. But in 2003, during the 3rd world congress of the Global Osteoarthritis Research Network (GORN) Pr Steven Abramson from the University of New York demonstrated that in osteoarthritis the joint is damaged since it is subjected to the pro-inflammatory affects of substances called cytokines. Where do they come from? They are generated by cartilage cells themselves or the synovial fluid surrounding the joint. Once synthesized they encourage cartilage cells to continue to produce them. This is when the inflammation becomes chronic.

Joints, the targets of osteoarthritis

Osteoarthritis only affects the ankle, elbow and wrist when these joints have been injured. It mainly strikes the knees, hips and vertebrae. For a simple reason of weight: these are the support points the body rests on.

The knees

This is osteoarthritisis' favorite joint! Often there is no symptom: thus osteoarthritis is diagnosed by chance or when a joint locks. But in most cases, the pain, changing, whimsical, minor in the beginning, becomes more and more bothersome. It is normally located on the front of the knee and moves downward due to the progressive alteration of the joint between the leg bones (tibia and fibula) and the kneecap. Going up or down stairs, walking on uneven ground, squatting, sitting for a long time, all becomes trying. On the contrary, walking on flat ground is painless. It is important to note that pain in the knee may actually be coming from the hip. This always needs to be examined when there is a complaint (*read below*).

The hips

Our hips support all of our weight with each step. The pain is generally located at the fold of the groin, the region which connects the thigh to the trunk, and sometimes on the outer side or in the buttock. It can extend along the thigh, reaching the knee. Walking and rotating movements hurt; it becomes difficult to put on your socks, pull up hose or bend

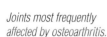

Joints most frequently affected by osteoarthritis.

over to wash your feet. In one person out of ten, osteoarthritis of the hip does not evolve: the pain remains but the joint continues to work. When cartilage deterioration is extreme, a prosthesis must be used (this is the case after an average of ten years). Osteoarthritis very frequently. reaches the second hip.

The vertebrae

All of the vertebrae can be affected, but the cervical and lumbar are those most affected. It is the disk which connects each vertebra in order to facilitate movements and absorb shocks, which suffers. And actually, too often we carry heavy objects without paying attention to our backs. And over time this joint also wears out and causes pain. In addition, the vertebrae alter to adapt and the nerves protruding from the spine are often compressed and thus the source of new pain. And this is why a bad back is called the disease of the century. An undoubtedly exaggerated expression but which is a reality! It is necessary to admit that the back, which is constantly strained, is severely tested. And we don't take care of it at all. Who always stands up straight? Who is careful to move slowly, and not stay in a bad position for too long? Or sleeps on their side, with one knee bent? Regular exercise helps develop back and abdominal muscles: they help you stand up straight and minimize the role of the back. We'll explain this all in detail later on.

The main risk factors

- Age
- Sex (females are more afflicted)
- Heredity
- Joint shocks and traumas
- Being overweight or obese
- Poor position and heavy loads
- Inflammatory diseases

I'm fed up with my hands!

10% of people over age 50 (mainly females) have osteoarthritis of the fingers. This is often hereditary. The fingers are swollen and sometimes painful. It is the distal phalanx (the one closest to the nail) which is more likely to deform than the proximal phalanx (closer to the hand). It often becomes more and more difficult to write, to use your fingers for a long time or for precise movements. The more you age, the greater the number of diseased joints. Osteoarthritis is also very frequent in the back of the hands. The pain is mitigated by decreasing mobility.

Everyone has osteoarthritis!

60 million people are diagnosed with osteoarthritis in the US each year. A disease as old as the world which strikes women more than men.

A widespread disease

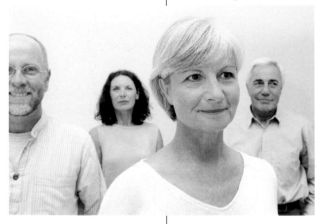

Osteoarthritis, is a disease which has always afflicted humans: skeletons found of our ancestor *homo sapiens* demonstrate this. So, in the elderly, osteoarthritis is a normal phenomenon, tied to aging of the body. Around 90% of people over age 65 suffer from it. But osteoarthritis can also occur in younger individuals, for different reasons: 9 % of people aged 21 are afflicted with the disease. In this case it is an osteoarthritis linked to traumas or after a joint operation. Osteoarthritis affects 17% of the population, regardless of age. Based on figures obtained from the French national health institute and a medical study on 145,000 employees from the French electricity company (GAZEL cohort) over several years, 14% of people aged 30 to 50 have osteoarthritis. Data from an American study made it possible to clarify the frequency of manifestations since osteoarthritic can damage joints without any pain or inflammation. Only 3% of people between the ages of 45 and 54 feel pain from osteoarthritis. One the other hand, 15% of those between 65 and 74 complain of pain. Osteoarthritis is a chronic disease which evolves over the years and whose signs vary greatly from one person to the next.

Women are more affected than men

After age 55, women are often more affected than men. They represent 2 patients out of 3. This vulnerability may be linked to osteoporosis, a process which weakens the bones due to hormonal upheavals during menopause. The bones of the joints may also be more fragile, and don't contribute to proper functioning of the joints. In addition, an American study demonstrated that women are more seriously affected than men. At the same age or after the same number of years with the disease, their joints are more damaged than men's. The number of afflicted joints is also higher. The causes of this have not yet been clearly established: hormonal? Genetic, tied to the female sex?

When the disease evolves

Osteoarthritis takes hold progressively. It sometimes evolves in spurts and the cartilage becomes softer and weaker and is destroyed. The joint is particularly stiff, swollen, red and at these times, the pain becomes more persistent. After several years, the pain manifests differently. It occurs more frequently, at any time of the day and lasts longer. It starts to be bothersome at night as well. The adjacent muscles may become sensitive or even painful.

The first signs of osteoarthritis

No matter what the sex, the first signs of osteoarthritis appear between the ages of 50 and 60. In the first months or first years, pain occurs during physical exertion or if too much effort is exerted. Later, it tends to manifest as soon as fatigue is felt. In some individuals it occurs at the end of the day: the joints are painful at night when it is time to go to sleep but not in the morning or the middle of the night.

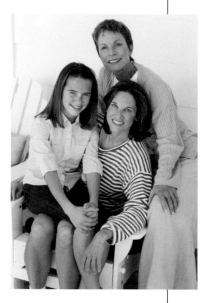

Osteoarthritic risk factors

Everyone has osteoarthritis because cartilage degeneration is mainly linked to age. However, certain factors increase the risk of getting this disease.

There are 3 major groups of risk factors:
- genetic factors: these are determined when we are born. They come from the genes of our parents but also from accidents or an infection during pregnancy. They are congenital anomalies:

- acquired factors, which correspond to events occurring during our life, like aging or weight gain;

- environmental factors: these are related to work, sports, etc.

Genes which play tricks

LResearchers have demonstrated that the occurrence of osteoarthritis is linked to sex. After age 50, it is much more frequent in women than in men, primarily of the knee! A muscular weakness, mainly of the thigh muscle, is also responsible for osteoarthritis of the knee. Congenital diseases increase the risk of osteoarthritis as well, as frequently occurs in the hip... many elements are linked to genetic heredity. Genetic and acquired factors, include the hormonal state of women: the sex-hormone combination, that leads to trouble!

Women, more vulnerable after age 50

Women are protected by their sexual hormones, estrogen... until they reach menopause, when the level of these hormones drops sharply. This is why an upsurge of the disease is observed in women starting at age 50. To prevent osteoarthritis, such as osteoporosis, women should get regular exercise and follow a diet which is rich in calcium and balanced for their entire lives.

A life which wears out joints

Aging, obesity, hormonal state are hazards of life. Since we can't do anything about age, we should watch our weight. If obesity is avoided, this decreases osteoarthritis of the knee by 25 to 50% according to some researchers ! Age also plays a role in development of osteoarthritis: 52% of adults over age 75 have at least one affected joint! The more we age, the more the cartilage in our joints deteriorates, letting the disease take hold. Infections of the joints also destroy the joint if they are not treated in time. All conditions which affect the joints and bones may promote osteoarthritis. This is the case of

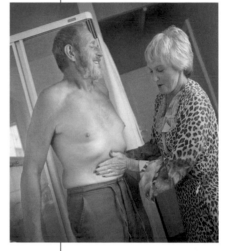

metabolic diseases, like gout. Surgery, with its risk of infection may also cause osteoarthritis. Knee operations in particular, may lead to osteoarthritis of the knee. Our environment also conceals some pitfalls: physical and professional occupations which involve repetitive movements, progressively wear out the joints. This involves workers, constructions workers, maintenance jobs, etc. Traumas and injuries to joints resulting from these jobs are also a frequent cause of osteoarthritis. Lastly, even spare time activities can lead to risks for our joints: gardening and somewhat violent sports. On the other hand, our diet can help us fight against osteoarthritis if we have a higher intake of vitamin C and D. This has been proven by recent studies.

Stress and a bad back

Even the psychological life and its hazards play a role! Shyness, nervousness, over-working or even stress can result in a bad back. A death, depression or even a conflict can result in physical weakness.

How do you know if you have osteoarthritis?

Painful joints, which are stiff in the morning and creak... these are telling signs. However, a physician's advice is necessary for establishing a correct diagnosis.

A disease which plays hide and seek

Osteoarthritis may remain hidden for a long time: pain only occurs after the cartilage destruction process has begun. Based on the amount of pain, the disease is divided into 4 stages:

Stade 1: the osteoarthritis exists but the person does not feel anything, doctors call it latent osteoarthritis (or asymptomatic osteoarthritis).

Stade 2: only pain is present, the other signs such as stiffness or creaking are not present yet (painful, unactivated osteoarthritis).

Stade 3: all of the symptoms of the disease are present (pain, stiffness, creaking). They say that the osteoarthritis is activated.

Stade 4: the disease becomes difficult to treat, occurrences multiply (decompensated osteoarthritis).

What should I tell my doctor?

If your joints are painful, your doctor will ask you to describe the pain: where does it hurt? Does the pain move? Is it very strong? Does it pull ? Does it throb? Do you have a hard time walking or climbing the stairs? Does the pain bother you so much that you have a hard time doing everyday tasks? Is your joint swollen or red, indicating an inflammation?

Also tell your doctor if you have recently run a temperature, have lost your appetite or lost weight. If this is the case, this information will most likely make him or her think it is arthritis, an inflammation of the joints. It is also important to say if your professional activity requires carrying heavy loads or if other members of your family have osteoarthritis or have undergone joint surgery.

At the end of this discussion, your doctor will take a look at your joints to understand the extent that the osteoarthritis is harming your mobility. If your knee is affected, the doctor

will examine your joint in 3 positions:
• standing up to look for any deformities in the joint;
• walking to evaluate any difficulties in moving and the need to use a cane;
• bent: certain movements are often painful. Twisting, when turning back around, for example, makes the the joint work under force. The doctor will reproduce this movement to "test" it.

What other examinations are necessary

An x-ray of the painful joint or joints is used to confirm the doctor's diagnosis. It can reveal several classical signs. An x-ray reflects the disease and changes in bones with a delay. There is no correspondence between the intensity of the pain and the importance of the x-ray findings: some lesions which are visible on an x-ray may not cause any harm. If there are questions a blood test may be necessary. The "sedimentation speed" and "C-reactive protein" level is measured to assess the amount of inflammation. The protein is released by the body as a reaction to an injury, infection or inflammation. It blood level systematically increases in the event of inflammation. In this case, the doctor excludes a simple osteoarthritis diagnosis.

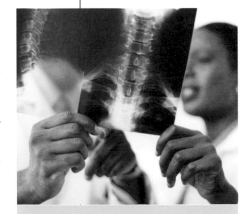

Understanding an x-ray in three words

On an x-ray, three major signs reveal osteoarthritis.

– Osteophytosis: the bones produce bony tissue to fight against joint destruction. Osteophytosis is better known by the name "parrot beaks".

– A decrease in the space between two bony surfaces, called "joint space" appears. This is the famous "narrow joint space".

– "Cysts" are areas of cartilage destruction which may spread to the joint when the evolution is significant. This also translates into affliction of the joint.

THE OTHER RHEUMATISMS

Deceptive diseases

All joint pain is not necessarily linked to classical osteoarthritis. Before age 45, it is necessary to be careful and have a complete check-up.

A lot of pain is called "projected": the person thinks the problem is where the pain is, when actually the source of the pain is elsewhere. This is the case, for example, of a pain in the buttock that one thinks is linked to the progressive destruction of the hip joint, but which, in reality, is due to pressure on a nerve. This is the case of "sciatica" which is pain in the buttock or along the thigh. Logically, the nerve which is pinched will be painful along its entire route. Sometimes the pain "stops" along the way and starts up later.

Inflammatory pain

Certain forms of osteoarthritis may have more of an inflammatory than mechanical aspect. During a worsening of the disease, there is an increase in the signs. In this case it is necessary to ensure that the affliction is purely mechanical in order to rule out arthritis, a joint inflammation. X-rays and a blood test can help the doctor to find a diagnosis and an adequate treatment. In some cases, the joint pain remains isolated, without any other sign. The x-rays do not contribute any information, nor does biology. The patient and doctor may both remain skeptical! Only evolution over time will

Sometimes even children are affected

Children are not spared from joint inflammation. 1 child out of 1000 suffers from chronic juvenile arthritis. This disease which affects one or more joints, starts before age 16. Its cause is unknown. It may disappear completely or occur in bouts. Fortunately, it is not a hereditary disease.

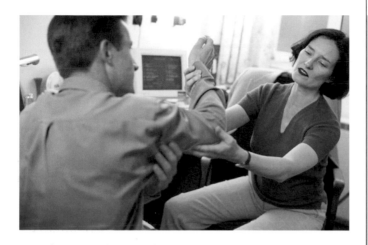

What is a "puncture"?
A puncture in a joint is part of a treatment performed when a joint is swollen, a sign of poor joint functioning. This is the case in certain diseases where the fluid present in the joint cavity is no longer reabsorbed. A thin needle is inserted in the swollen part to withdraw a little fluid. An analysis of the synovial fluid is used to obtain the information necessary for adapting the treatment. The puncture is also used to eliminate the joint swelling, thus to relieve the pain.

confirm the diagnosis of steoarthritis. So it is necessary to treat the pain first.

Other signs of inflammation

The pain rarely remains isolated. Fever and fatigue are often associated. It may also be accompanied by an effusion. This swelling of the joint is connected to a change in the synovial tissue which no longer correctly plays its role as a sponge for the synovial fluid. The swollen joint becomes more and more difficult to bend or extend. A puncture is necessary. to drain the fluid.

Osteoarthritis or arthritis?

Two opposite afflictions of the joint: osteoarthritis which has a mechanical cause (trauma, aging of the bones, etc.) and arthritis which is an inflammation of the joint. The pain does not occur at the same time (the evening for osteoarthritis, the night for arthritis). A blood test can be used to diagnose the inflammation. A x-ray can be used to tell the difference. And lastly, a puncture in the joint, if it is swollen from fluid, does not have the same results.

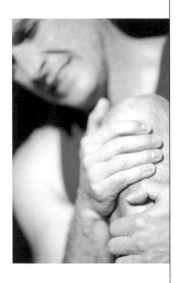

Infectious arthritis: when germs attack

Germs may be at the origin of joint pain. Infectious arthritis is more likely to affect people who already have weak joints.

Infectious arthritis is more likely to affect major joints such as the shoulder, hip or knee. Fingers or the ankles are less likely to be affected. These are viruses or bacteria which cause the destruction of the cartilage. This destruction of cartilage, called necrosis, starts an inflammation. The joint becomes sensitive and a little warm, slightly swollen and red. This is a sign that the body is reacting and fighting back. Sometimes, the inflammatory reaction is enough to resist the germ attack. Thus the cartilage is not too damaged and the infection has no other repercussions. Unfortunately in most cases, the inflammation last too long and goes beyond its initial role of protecting the joint. If it goes untreated or is treated too

How do germs get into the joint?

Certain situations increase the risk of developing an infection. These include:

People with a weak immune system;

- diabetics;
- alcoholics;
- people with rheumatoid arthritis;
- people who have been taking corticosteriods for a long time.

late, the joint is invaded by germs, the inflammation spreads and there may be serious consequences, including complete destruction of the joint. An infection of the adjacent joint may then develop and in the most serious cases spread throughout the body. There are no mistaking the signs of inflammation: the joint becomes very red and hot and, more importantly, the pain becomes worse and worse, accompanied by fever and chills.

Suitable antibiotics

The main germs responsible for arthritis are staphylococci, accounting for more than 60%. More rarely, the tuberculosis bacteria may affect the joints, like viruses or parasites. It is important to know the origin of the microbe in order to be able to correctly treat the inflammation with antibiotics. Each antibiotic is specific for one or more bacteria. This is why you sometimes here "antibiotics, aren't good for anything!". This is actually the case if they are given indiscriminately, when the microbe has not been identified. Joint lavages performed using a probe filled with saline solution, are used to deeply clean the infected joint. Then, in addition to the medications, it is very important to mobilize the affected joint as soon as possible, so that it does not become numb.

How do germs get into the joint?

Microbes, or germs, include bacteria, viruses and parasites. They can infect a joint in three ways:
• Microbes can spread in the entire body when they reach the blood vessels and the joints they normally do not escape because they are vascularized.
• An operation on a joint, even if performed in a sterile environment, runs the risk of a microbe entering the body.
• A trauma may cause a deep enough injury for a microbe to be able to enter a joint.

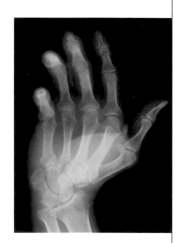

Rheumatoid arthritis

Osteoarthritis is not the only disease to affect joints. And all joint disorders are not necessarily rheumatisms, a term often used ill-advisably.

In rheumatoid arthritis, it is the immune system which attacks the synovial tissue lining the joint bone. The inflammation mainly effects the small joints of the limbs, i.e. the fingers, toes and wrists. Generally both side of the body are affected at the same time. The hips, shoulders or the joints of the head and neck can also be swollen and painful. Rheumatoid arthritis is three times more frequent in women. It can occur at any age, with a peak between age 30 and 50. A Dutch study pointed to drinking coffee as a cause, without really reaching a conclusion. On the other hand, the disease is less likely to affect those who suffer from hay fever, and those who regularly eat cooked vegetables, olive oil and supplements containing zinc.

Significant signs

This disease starts out with very general symptoms. Fatigue, loss of appetite, weight loss, or even the sweating that it causes do not make it possible to identify it immediately. It really starts when one or more joints start to swell. They then become painful and stiff, especially in the morning. Strength in the hands and fingers starts to decrease. Symptoms similar to those of arthritis then begin: a simple pain at night and in the morning at the beginning, then the appearance of redness and a

What are the causes?

There are many causes for this disease. From samples of bone marrow studies have been conducted demonstrating that genetic factors certainly play a role. A hormonal origin is also plausible: a recurrence of the disease is often observed during pregnancy, a time when the body is filled with hormones.

sensation of heat after a few months. As the disease evolves, it becomes more and more difficult to make accurate movements. The affected joints deform and sometimes the adjacent muscles decrease in volume. The hands, fingers and feet deform in a very typical manner, called "claw toes" or even "ulnar deviation" for the hand.

An unpredictable future

The evolution is extremely variable: between total and long-lasting remission (no more signs) and chronic and disabling aggravation, it is possible to see all the stages. All hope is therefore allowed! Anti-inflammatory drugs act against the pain and morning stiffness. It is also important to exercise to keep the joints in good shape and avoid bad positions. The joints speak for themselves: x-rays make it possible to more precisely assess the seriousness of the disorders. A blood test indicates other symptoms frequent with this disease: anemia, inflammation and low iron. It can also detect the "rheumatoid factor", an autoantibody characteristic of this disease found in around 80% of patients.

What is an autoimmune disease?

It is a disruption of the immune system, the system which protects the body. To protect itself against aggressors (microbes) the organism defends itself with antibodies.. In autoimmune diseases, it directs these antibodies against itself: these are called auto-antibodies.

Smokers, you are at greater risk

Tobacco is a well-known risk factor for this disease. For 10 years, American researchers followed 31,336 women aged 55 to 69 living in Iowa. Women who smoke have a 2 times higher risk of rheumatoid arthritis compared to women who have never smoked. The higher and longer the consumption of tobacco the higher the risk.

Gout

Gout attacks start when uric acid is deposited abnormally in the joints. The pain is similar to that of arthritis.

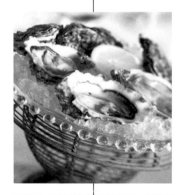

Living with gout

People who are afflicted with gout attacks must take a break in the country in order to prevent them. A diet free from shellfish, game and offal is recommended. Eating meat, poultry and fish should be limited. It is also advisable to avoid alcohol. Being over-weight or obese is often tied to high levels of uric acid in the blood. Losing weight may also make it possible to limit the disease.

Gout is caused by an excess of uric acid in the blood. It then gets into the joints but also into the tissue under the skin and at times even the kidneys. Uric acid is a substance which causes the destruction of "nucleic acids", a type of genetic link which makes up our DNA (genetic heritage). The constant renewal of our cells thus makes its presence normal in the blood. Uric acid is also produced during digestion of foods rich in nucleic acids, such as offal, shellfish or even game. Food-caused gout accounts for less than 10% of cases. Often, the real cause cannot be found. Gout may be a side effect of certain medications (for example for tuberculosis) or even caused by kidney failure. It is the kidneys which filter blood and thus regulate uric acid by eliminating any excess through urine.

A very male disease

Gout attacks primarily start around age 45 but can even begin at age 20. They mainly effect men who represent 90 to 95 % of cases. In women, the first signs only appear after menopause. Women actually have a lower level of uric acid than men, which is why they are less vulnerable. Gout attacks usually occur at night with an abrupt, violent pain, most of the time in a joint. This is very inflammatory: red, swollen and painful. The joint which is most often affected is located at the base of the big toe. But it may also affect the ankles, knees and even the wrists or fingers; several joints may be affected at the same time. The attacks usually occur after eating brain, liver, kidney, seafood or game. Drinking alcohol decreases the elimination of uric acid. Infections, even an accident can trigger the attacks. Between two attacks, the presence of synovial fluid in the joint is not rare.

Medications

Doctors only prescribe medication when the attacks become more and more frequent (more than 3 attacks per year) or if the kidneys are affected by deposits. Colchicine, a specific anti-inflammatory drug, is used to treat the attacks. It is a medication which increases the uric acid eliminated by the kidneys. A medication which blocks the synthesis of uric acid is used to treat people whose disease is genetic in origin (the body produces too much uric acid.)

Microcrystalline arthritis

Gout and chondrocalcinosis are part of what are called "microcrystalline arthritis". This name comes from the origin of these diseases. Small particles,microcrystals deposit on the joints, blocking their normal functioning.

The different forms of the disease

There are different forms of gout: the rarest ones are characterized by the presence of "tophus": this is a deposit of uric acid in the skin and bones, which only appears in very severe evolutions of the disease. In other cases, it is simply an arthritis without the famous tophus.

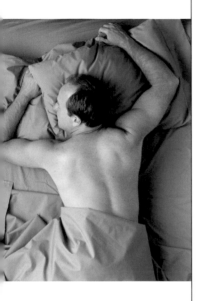

Ankylosing spondylitis

Ankylosing spondylitis is a form of arthritis which affects the spine. It is a chronic condition, associated with inflammation and rheumatisms.

Ankylosing spondylitis starts between the end of adolescence and age 40. Young men, between the ages of 18 and 35, are the most affected. Actually, 9 times more males than females suffer from this disease and the reason remains unknown. 1% of the population is affected. The origin of this complex disease is unknown. According to British researchers, those with the disease have high levels of an antibody called lgA, which may be a sign of an immune system reaction to a colon bacteria.

Spondylitis first affects the pelvic bones and the lower part of the spine. More rarely, the heel, hip or knee. In the beginning, the symptoms of the disease are very vague and above all common. The person complains of pain starting at the buttock and moving down the leg. He or she feels stiff and is often woken up by lumbar pain or in the legs. Bouts of fever, weight loss and fatigue indicate surges of the inflammation.

The pain increases over time. It becomes difficult to move and bend. The back is actually stiffer and stiffer and tilted. This is what is called "bamboo spine". It is straight like bamboo and has the same "stripes" on an x-ray, due to changes in the bones.

A very strange risk factor

Scientific studies have shown that the same genetic factor is present in 90% of people affected by ankylosing spondylitis. Only 8% of the population in good health is a carrier of this genetic factor called "HLA B27".

And after, how do you live a normal life?

Various examinations, particularly x-rays are required to diagnose ankylosing spondylitis.

The "bamboo spine" is a key diagnostic element. Blood tests indicate an inflammation: the sedimentation rate and C-reactive protein (CRP) increase. Once a diagnosis is made, it is necessary to treat the disease and learn how to live with it. Anti-inflammatory drugs are used to relieve inflammations and pain. If the disease gets worse, a stronger treatment with an immunosuppressant drug is given. Lifestyle is very important. A diet low in spices, alcohol and chocolate decreases the side effects of these drugs on the stomach. Phytotherapy (meadowsweet, horseweed, white willow, blackcurrant and harpagophytum) is also very interesting. When it is worse rest is indispensable. This is one of the keys of treatment. This must be done on the back, on a hard surface, without a pillow, in order not to increase deformities. Physical therapy (teaching our body certain postures and movements) is essential in this disease. This is done with the assistance of a physical therapist, sometimes in a pool. If the back deformity is significant, wearing a corset may be necessary.

Sports help!

Just because you are sick doesn't mean you need to stop moving! Quite the opposite, sports are really beneficial. Violent sports, like combat sports or tennis are not recommended. On the other hand, swimming on your stomach is particularly recommended. Finally, if your condition is worse, it is best to refrain from all physical exercise.

The experience of Dr Seignalet

In his book *L'alimentation ou la troisième médecine*, Dr Jean Seignalet (Montpellier) showed how the modern diet has negative effects on our health ... but also how specific diets may be the key to healing. The diet mainly consists in eliminating all cereals (except rice and buckwheat) animal milk, and to eat a maximum of raw vegetables (organic) virgin vegetable oils and to take vitamin and mineral supplements. If the diet is followed closely, after 1 year, 96% of patients suffer less and recovery mobility.

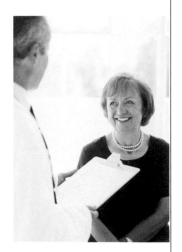

FROM THE DOCTOR TO THE OSTEOPATH, WHO DOES WHAT?

What physicians should be consulted ?

Treating osteoarthritis falls under various medical: disciplines, surgery and physical therapy are the most frequent.

Family physician

Your family doctor knows you well, so naturally you'd turn to him or her to discuss the pain that is disabling you during everyday life. He or she is the most capable of diagnosing a problem and treating it. It will be easy for him or her to tell you if you have osteoarthritis.

If it is difficult to make a diagnosis, he or she will have you take additional tests or refer you to a rheumatologist. Family doctors often have to deal with patients affected with osteoarthritis, the most frequent disease of the elderly. And since the overall age of population is increasing, the frequency of the disease is on the rise. Thus doctors are becoming more and more capable of effectively handling your problems. It is extremely beneficial to be followed by the same person. This person, based on his or her knowledge of your body and the evolution of your disease, can best adapt the treat-

Injections, specialty of rheumatologists

Rheumatologists are the most qualified doctors for giving injections. These are local shots given in the painful joint. They involve injecting corticosteroids exactly into the painful place. These drugs relieve inflammation and thus pain for a few weeks, up to a maximum of two months. Afterwards, their effectiveness decreases.

ment. You should know that for all chronic diseases, and not just osteoarthritis, regular follow-up and with the same doctor, is highly recommended. He or she is your ideal contact on a day-to-day basis and is the easiest to consult.

Rheumatology specialists

Doctors are divided into two categories: general practitioners who treat all the pathologies of the population, and specialists who concentrate on an organ (cardiology, for the heart) or a part of the population (geriatrics for the elderly, pediatrics). Rheumatologists dedicate themselves to the study and treatment of diseases of the bones and joints, i.e. what is called the musculoskeletal system. They also treat muscles, tendons and ligaments. Just like general practitioners, they can prescribe anti-inflammatory medications, painkillers and others. They perform injections or manipulations. Few doctors are authorized to do this: it involves moving the various bone structures in relation to each other, in order to but them back in the correct position. This treatment is slightly "violent", thus it is necessary to perfectly know the anatomy of the human body in order not to worsen the pain instead of making it better! Rheumatologists also treat all of the factors involved with osteoarthritis: stress, nutrition and triggering factors, which should not be neglected in favor of manipulation. They will also prescribe physical therapy sessions for you to perform at a physical therapist in order to restore all movements and flexibility to the joint.

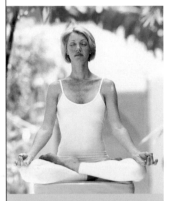

Yoga by the Yogi

Yogi Babacar Khane is an osteopath and chiropractor. He collaborated closely with the famous rheumatologist Philippe Baumgartner. He was later able to develop effective yoga techniques for the prevention and treatment of numerous rheumatology diseases. Yoga acts in two ways: on one hand, by making movements so that the joints work, on the other through the relaxation and well-being that you feel during the sessions. It is not greatly racticed, but courses and training are proposed on the website devoted to Y. B. Khane.

Orthopedic surgeons and the family doctor

Orthopedic surgeons get involved when it is time to operate. Physiatrists are helpful when it is time to recover motor functions.

When the joint break down

Orthopedic surgeons are obviously surgeons. Generally, people who have a fracture, deformities or diseases of the skeleton consult this specialist. Your doctor will refer you to one if you need to be fitted with a prosthesis. Sometimes in cases of advanced osteoarthritis, medications are no longer sufficient for treating the patient's pain. When all other solutions turn out to be ineffective, it is best to operate and insert a prosthesis to replace the defective joint. Orthopedic surgeons follow their patients for the entire course of the operation: beforehand, they make a diagnosis making sure it is necessary to operate. Then they operate and fit the prosthesis. Lastly, they take care of the necessary prescriptions after the operation and the indispensable rehabilitation. It is necessary to know whether to consult an orthopedic surgeon when you have too much pain and medications are ineffective. He or she will be able to tell you if your problem can be treated with surgery, and if not, he or she can refer you to another doctor.

Let's go, on your feet!

After a complete knee prosthesis operation, rehabilitation makes it possible to walk normally again as quickly as possible. To start pulleys are used to gently move your leg. Then with a splint for support, you can stand up 4 days after the operation. After a week you'll walk with a cane. And after 3 weeks you'll take on the stairs!

Physiatrists: pros and cons

Physical medicine is for a long time in the United States considered as a recognized specialization. This type of medical practice was finally accepted in France at the beginning of the 1970's. These specialists treat all orthopedic, rheumatology, neurological or even respiratory pathologies: they all require special rehabilitation. There are different forms of of treatment: physiatrists perform manipulations, manual therapies and mobilizations. The sometimes use different devices to complete the therapy: lasers, electrical currents or temperature working with cold. They also use hydrotherapy (read page 68). Exercise and massages may be effective. However, you need to be careful: some physiatrists often rely solely on manipulations, sometimes performed too quickly. The treatment they propose to you needs to work for you and, more importantly, give you relief.

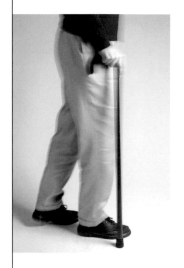

Prostheses from A to Z

Prostheses can replace all joints: wrist, ankle and even the phalanx! Nevertheless, prostheses of the knee and hip are the most frequent. They represent more than 60% of all fitted prostheses! Many men and women benefit from these operations which are mainly performed on those over age 65. Prostheses can be set, a type of "glue" fixes the prosthesis like a stamp on an envelop, or held by a plate screwed on the bone. Currently, three different materials are used: metal, plastic or ceramic.

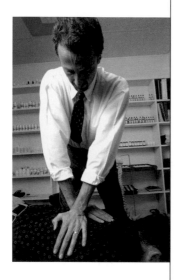

Not doctors but indispensable all the same!

More or less controversial, between standardized maneuvers and more obscure tactics, here is a presentation of the other remaining players! Their role is just as important as that of doctors and their effectiveness may prove to be pertinent.

Physical therapist

Physical therapists follow 3 or 4 years of specialization in this discipline. They know all the human body's muscles and anatomy perfectly. They have perfect mastery of rehabilitation techniques for operated or injured patients. The doctor prescribes the actions performed by the physical therapist. This may involve massages, application of heat or electrical currents, rehabilitation techniques or even mobilizations. Attention: physical therapists are not trained for performing manipulations. They work in partnership with doctors since their respective treatments are complementary. The contribute an indispensable aide to patient recovery. It is necessary to admit that doctors do not always exactly know the precise physical therapy techniques and rely on the skill of the physical therapists. They give them rather vague instructions in terms of practical performance, but very exact ones concerning the results to obtain and functions to improve. Physical therapists know how to relieve and massage their patients. They mobilize failing joints in order to recover their function. Step by step, thanks to physical therapy sessions, simple everyday actions like climbing the stairs or going out in the yard become easier and less painful.

Osteopaths

Osteopathy is a real hotbed of controversy, both regarding the recognition of osteopaths in France, and on repayment for their examinations and even education. Let's take a closer look! Osteopathy originated in the United States in 1874. It quickly took hold in England ...the opposite of France where it was only recognized as a separate specialization starting February 19, 2002. After long debates between doctors and physical therapists, a decision was made that "all French individuals in possession of a high school diploma and who have followed a course authorized by the government may practice osteopathy". Based on osteopathy theories, a mechanical disorder or affected joint is responsible for pathological manifestations. They may be related to the bones, muscles, nerves, ligaments or vascular. They are the cause of "functional" diseases, i.e. psychological, or even organic. This is where the osteopath acts, mainly with body manipulations. Attention, osteopathy is often considered as manipulation, but this is not its only way of treating. The fee for a consultation if generally around 50 dollars for a 45 minute session. The National Public Health Service does not reimburse the fee and only some insurance companies will pick up part of the charge. It is best to find out about this beforehand.

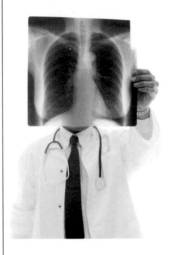

WHAT ARE THE SOLUTIONS FOR TREATING OSTEOARTHRITIS?

Everyday living with osteoarthritis

It is well known that for someone affected by osteoarthritis, each movement can be painful and each deformity very unpleasant. But those who have never been ill, who have never suffered on a daily basis, how do they know how someone feels?

Neglected pain and depression

Suffering for some individuals is a fatality. It is normal to become somewhat used to suffering. But after a certain amount of time, it is your mind which will pay! Daily pain can cause depression which in turn increases the pain. Things exist to give you relief, you shouldn't forget this and above all do not hesitate to talk about it.

24 hours of the life of a patient

Frances is 70 years old. Osteoarthritis has been part of her life for a long time. She is a very dynamic person, and decided that neither her age nor her osteoarthritis would run her life. So, she accepted her pain and learned how to manage things day to day. When she wakes up it is very difficult for her to move flexibly and easily. Just getting out of bed causes pain in the lumbar area; however she needs to go and get her breakfast! Frances does not want to take a lot of medications for a long time: she goes for physical therapy treatment every day which she has had to abandon two or three times a year during stronger osteoarthritis attacks, to take anti-inflammatory drugs. Opening a door is an ordeal in the morning: it is a painful flash which pierces her elbow. Moreover, she loved to write and has been forced to renounce her favorite hobby since her thumb can't handle it: this joint is also effected by the erosion of cartilage and bone. Walking is also painful when she gets up. No more quick trips to the bakery and grocery store early in the morning: when her foot assumes a certain position when she walks, it feels like she is being stabbed in the back. So, unfortunately for her, it is much more pleasant and easier to go out later in the morning. Actually, Frances has noticed that after an hour, she no longer has the feeling of being "stiff": she now knows that the "morning loosening up" is mandatory!

Day to day

The daytime is better: the pain lessens, even if it is still present, like a slightly muted discomfort. It is always located in the same places (mainly the thumbs, elbows, lumbar and top of the foot). And no day is like the previous one: she needs to adapt based on her shape. The ability to adapt is indispensable for correctly managing her disease: she needs to take things as they come. To acquire a certain philosophy... Fortunately, in the evening there is no recurrence. She should sleep flat but this is not always necessary. In this case, it is not rare to sleep in a poor position, on one side. And then, waking up is even more painful. But the worst pain for Frances was an attack of sciatica linked to pressure on nerve roots caused by osteoarthritis bone spurs. These nerves projecting from the spinal cord are slightly crushed by the bony growth. They trigger pain which is very difficult to withstand. It starts from the buttock and travels along the thigh (on the outside) then the calf and lastly, under the foot to the big toe. Finally, this is just a bad memory for her.

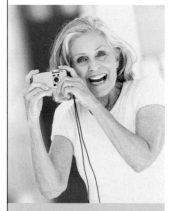

Move around and travel!

Frances continues to lead an active life and travel: her doctor told her that physical activity, without overdoing it, is part of osteoarthritis treatment. It acts like a "rust-remover" on mechanical parts. Stretching exercises are also recommended since they help muscles and their relearning their role to support the joint. Life can be very beautiful, even with osteoarthritis!

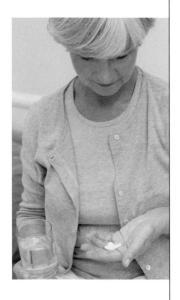

Conquering and treating pain

Painkillers are prescribed to treat the joints and all forms of pain and inflammation. The substances used vary based on the intensity of the pain. Explanations, from acetaminophen to morphine...

Painkillers are very standardized. There are non-morphine painkillers and morphine painkillers. In the latter group, there are those which act against a fever (antipyretic), like acetaminophen, and anti-inflammatory drugs (aspirin). Sold over the counter, without a prescription, acetaminophen is the main painkiller. It is used to relieve all pain (tooth, joint, headache, etc.). And it is highly effective against rheumatic pain. Similar to aspirin, but without anti-inflammatory properties, it is better to use when it is sufficient for controlling the pain. It acts on the brain, is not addicting and does not have side effects (except for allergies).

Anti-inflammatory drugs

These are the second most used medication for treating rheumatisms. In addition to an analgesic action, it acts on the inflammation. Thus it is a benchmark for osteoarthritis, once acetaminophen is no longer sufficient. Aspirin fights against pain and inflammation. It also thins the blood. The only problem is its side effects: it is harmful for the stomach and may cause hemorrhages or allergies. Other anti-inflammatory drugs, like ibuprofen (Nurofen®) or "coxibs" are also interesting for treating osteoarthritis, since they have fewer effects on the stomach. However, it is important to know that one of the coxibs, rofecoxib (Vioxx) increases the risk of heart

attacks and strokes. This has been observed after continuous treatment for 18 months (which is the opposite
of anti-inflammatory drug prescriptions, particularly in
osteoarthritis). Rofecoxib has been withdrawn from the
market but now uncertainty persists regarding the other
coxibs even if no study has demonstrated that they
increase the risk of heart attacks and strokes.

Morphine and its derivatives

Lastly, at the very top of the painkiller range is morphine.
Morphine acts on the central nervous system (brain and
spinal cord), and this is how it controls the routes of the
pain. But its side effects are far from being minor and may
be difficult to withstand. This is why it is reserved for into-
lerable pain and is not usually used with osteoarthritis.

And during pregnancy?

Anti-inflammatory drugs are completely contraindicated during pregnancy. This is particularly true in the last three months since they can have a dangerous effect on the fetus' heart.

Generics: advantages and disadvantages

A generic is a drug which can replace a better known drug given for a disease. It is composed of the same chemical molecule, and thus contains the same active ingredient ...and thus has the same effectiveness. It is just as safe as its "big brother" but around 30% cheaper, since it is a copy of a medi- cation invented 20 years beforehand. This is actually the amount of time necessary for a patent to cease protecting the discovery of a new molecule. This is a very good thing for patients and the public health system! The only problem some doctors attribute to them is the possibility of side effects due to certain excipients, the substances used to "package" the active ingredient.

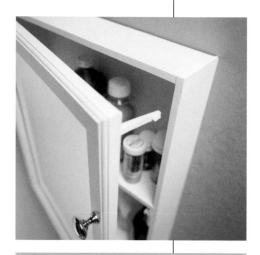

Side effects, the flip side of the coin?

Medications are taken to treat pain but sometimes they cause minor problems even ...real illnesses.

A medication that is harmful?

To treat a disease researchers try to determine an active ingredient which only acts on the diseased organ. But it triggers a cascade of chemical reactions, not all controlled and sometimes dangerous. Thus anti-inflammatory drugs often cause **digestion problems**, which are directly related to the way these medications act. The problems may range from simple burning to an ulcer or a major inflammation which can end up with hemorrhages and perforations of the stomach walls. According to studies, people who regularly take anti-inflammatory drugs have a 3-5 times higher risk of acquiring a stomach disease than those who don't take them. The esophagus and the intestines are not spared either. The stomach is characterized by its acidity, which helps digestion and lets it work better. The mucous membrane which lines the inside of the stomach is very fragile. It is protected by substances called prostaglandins. The anti-inflammatory drugs cause a decrease in the production of these protective substances which are indispensable for the stomach. Thus the mucous membrane is easily exposed to the aggression of the medications.

A life-preserver for the stomach

If you have a delicate stomach due to one of the following reasons, taking anti-inflammatory drugs must be accompanied by a medication that protects the stomach. This is the case if:

• you take numerous medications such as corticosteroids;

• you get heartburn;

• you get gastric reflux;

• you have had an ulcer ;

• you are affected by complications: perforation or hemorrhage of the stomach.

And the rest of the body?

• **The skin** is the second place that shows side effects after the stomach: hives, a desire to scratch or sudden redness on the face may appear after taking an anti-inflammatory drug. These signs are not serious. Anti-inflammatory drugs may sometimes go much further with serious dermatological diseases.

• **The kidneys** may also suffer from taking these drugs. In a healthy, young person who drinks enough there is no problem. But in the elderly, diabetics or people with a kidney disorder, the filtering role of the kidneys may be greatly altered due to anti-inflammatory drugs. This translates into high blood pressure, edemas (swelling of tissue due to water retention) or even heart failure or a kidney which no longer works correctly.

• **The heart** is not spared but only in very particular circumstances. Heart attacks have increased very slightly with the "coxibs" (one of the three classes of anti-inflammatory drugs). Other studies need to be conducted to confirm this observation.

However, in concluding this chapter we would like to reiterate that given the frequency with which anti-inflammatory drugs are prescribed, there are very few severe effects. The medications are often correctly prescribed and patients carefully monitored.

Also in your blood

Abnormalities may also appear in the blood when taking anti-inflammatory drugs:
• anemia (lack of red blood cells);
• lower platelet count (which plays a role in clotting and thus the repair of of wounds);
• lower white blood cell count (thus an increase in infections).
The liver can also be affected to a varying degree, sometimes even leading to hepatitis.

Injections

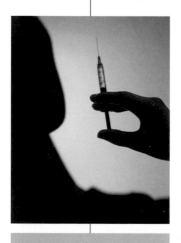

This very interesting technique is used to relieve pain. It involves injecting corticosteroids into the joint.

The examination is simple: the doctor inserts a needle into the joint, avoiding the tendons, veins or nerves. There are precise marking techniques used to be very familiar with anatomy ...and not pick the wrong place! For this reason, this procedure can only be performed by a doctor, either a general practitioner or a specialist. The injection may be painful: this is a momentary pain due to touching a nerve or an innervated element. It is like an electrical shock. But it does not always hurt! And you can't forget the very encouraging results on osteoarthritis or arthritis. The injection must be made in sterile conditions. A maximum of 3 to 4 injections per year are recommended. If two injections are necessary to get rid of the pain, there must be a four week interval between them. Corticosteroids have a delayed action equivalent to 3 or 4 weeks.

Corticosteroids

Corticosteroids are natural hormones secreted by the adrenal glands (located above the kidneys), after numerous transformations of cholesterol... Artificially synthesized, corticosteroid drugs are identical to natural hormones. They are used for their anti-inflammatory effect in the form of tablets (like cortisone), ointment or gel to apply to painful joints, or as a liquid to inject in joints or or muscles.

Relieving pain

The sole role of the injection is to relieve pain, thanks to the corticosteroids, when classic anti-inflammatory drugs no longer work. They do not cure osteoarthritis, arthritis or even an inflammation of the tendons, where they are also used to treat pain. And the effect of corticosteroids does not last forever! Corticosteroids act for a few weeks or months: this is still an important respite for someone who continually suffers. However, injections may not work for some people. You doctor can give you good advice on the choices you have between different treatments. Injections can be given in all joints. The amount of corticosteroids depends on the size of the joint to treat: it can range from a finger to a hip or from a knee to a wrist.

"Viscosupplementation"

Recently, hyaluronic acid injections have begun to be used as well. This substance is naturally present in the synovial fluid surrounding a joint. During osteoarthritis, the hyaluronic acid begins to disappear from this fluid. To overcome this shortage, the rheumatologist may perform "viscosupplementation", i.e. hyaluronic acid injections. This technique is very interesting for moderate osteoarthritis with little inflammation. Generally, the doctor makes 3 to 5 injections, one week apart. The hyaluronic acid works for 6 to 12 months or even longer. It acts by increasing the viscosity of the synovial fluid which limits rubbing between the cartilaginous surfaces and stimulates cartilage repair. Hyaluronic acid is very well tolerated. The only disadvantages: its cost (115 to 350 dollars for three injections) and the lack of feedback on its long-term effectiveness.

Dr Jekkyl and Mister Hide

Corticosteroids are fantastic medications in terms of their effectiveness... but they also have many side effects. They decrease immunity and thus increase infections. They harm the stomach and may be responsible for ulcers. They contribute to the loss of certain elements like potassium. And this ion is extremely important for the correct balance of the body. In conclusion, the less you take, the better it is!

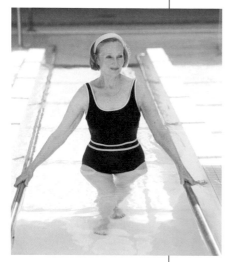

Physical therapy

Physical therapy sessions with a physical therapist help preserve or restore joint mobility and also relieve pain.

Straight ahead

If you suffer from **cervical or lumbar osteoarthritis**, the first goal of physical therapy is to decompress the joint to relieve pain. It can also be used to correct your posture in order to eliminate bending of the neck or lower back and stretch the spine. Generally, a session starts by applying heat (infrared or hot mud) and massages to relax and loosen the muscles.

Example of an exercise: standing against a wall, legs slightly bent and forward, put your hand in the curve of your lower back and head against the wall. Try to flatten your nape by completely pulling in the chin and stretching up, flatten the back by pressing your hands against the wall. Or on a mat on the ground, lie on your back, legs bent, feet flat on the floor and arms extended along your body. Try to make yourself taller as if gently pulling on a string hanging from the top of a crane, pulling in your chin and stomach.

Walking is great ...just don't overdo!

If you have **osteoarthritis of the knee or hip**, a golden rule: spare your joints. It is not unadvisable to uselessly strain your joints ....but that does not mean just letting them completely rest! Exercises greatly vary based on body weight. It is also recommended to lose a few pounds, the best solution for preserving the joint. The exercises are aimed at restoring the range necessary to the joint to be able to continue to walk normally. The muscles also need to work: toned, they stabilize the joint and ensure balance for the body. .

Example of an exercise: lie on your back, lift one leg and keep it completely straight (no bending your knee!) then hold it in this position or make small circles with the tip of your foot if you want. With the leg extended, tip of your foot pointing outwards, lift the leg diagonally above the other leg.

Careful, sudden unlocking!

To protect yourself and relieve pain when walking, the knee has some specific sensors, which sometimes send an order to the thigh muscles to release the contraction. If the muscle is weak, this fraction of a second is enough to suddenly unlock the knee joint. This is frequently the cause of falls in elderly people. Maintaining the quadriceps muscles of the thigh makes it possible to lock the knee and stay in a position with the leg outstretched. If the knee stays constantly bent while walking, the joint suffers excessively ...a process which reinforces osteoarthritis.

When the vertebrae fuse...

In elderly people, the cartilage damaged by osteoarthritis of the back, at cervical or lumbar level, cicatrizes in a bony form and causes the loss of mobility in the affected vertebrae, but this also signals the end of pain! In this stage, it must be avoided at all costs to let the vertebrae fuse into a poor position to limit the loss of mobility caused by the calcification to a minimum. It is advisable to lie, completely flat, on your stomach for at least 10 minutes a day (unless you have respiratory problems). You can put a small pillow under your stomach if the position is too painful.

In the water at... 35 °C!

If possible, choose a physical therapist who has access to a pool. Physical therapy in the water is often considered much more pleasant. The temperature, 35 °C (!), helps relieve pain. In the water, the hips and knees support less of the body's weight; it is also easier to work the arms, if you have cervical osteoarthritis. Only formal contraindications: high blood pressure and heart or circulation problems.

Is surgery a good solution?

When medications are no longer sufficient, it is possible to have an operation. First of all surgery can correct joint defects; at a more advanced stage, a prosthesis replaced a joint which is too damaged.

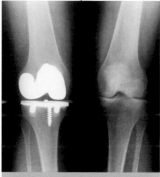

A brand new joint

There are two types of knee prosthesis. The entire knee joint can be replaced or a partial prosthesis can be put in the place where the cartilage is damaged. For the hips, there are only complete prostheses. Each year 1.000.000 people are operated.

First repair...

Due to the deformities it causes, osteoarthritis shatters the axis that exists between two bones. Instead of being correctly fitted to each other, they are no longer properly aligned to each other. This is where the surgeon intervenes. They correctly realign the joint. Thus the evolution of the disease is prevented or slowed down. Realigning the knee involves painful joints. This is possible in people under age 70. The ligaments around the joint must work well. An operation of this type makes it possible to delay fitting a knee prosthesis. For the hip joint, even younger people can be operated on, less than age 50. This is frequent for treating early osteoarthritis. Even just moderate discomfort is a good reason for operating. But unlike the knee, this type of operation will not prevent fitting a prosthesis.

My prosthesis, I'll protect it!

Right after the operation, the risk of phlebitis (a clot disturbing blood circulation) can be avoiding by resuming walking quickly. To prevent dislocation, sudden twisting movements towards the inside are forbidden, above all in the first 3 months after the operation. And long-term always consult your doctor immediately in the event of infection, even mild (tooth, bladder). Over time, the prosthesis may come loose: it goes out of alignment because it is no longer adapted to the bones it connects... but there is nothing you can do about it!

... and later possibly replace the joint

A realignment operation is not always enough to solve the disability caused by osteoarthritis. It is necessary in these cases to adopt a more radical treatment: fitting of a prosthesis. This decision is made by the surgeon based on the amount of pain and functional difficulties. Knee and hip prostheses are the most common, but there are also shoulder and ankle prostheses. More rarely, a prosthesis can be fitted for a disk between two vertebrae or a finger prosthesis. The wear of the material is inevitable, which is why prostheses need to be replaced. Prostheses last an average of 15 years. Changing a prosthesis when it gets old is an identical operation to the first one. It does not pose any problems, like the case before, unless, obviously, the health conditions of the patient jeopardize the operation. In older people, the decision is based on the person's mobility, their need to walk, and tolerance to pain. If the operation is not possible, a cane or wheelchair will let them preserve a certain amount of mobility.

And for osteoarthritis of the hand?

Surgery is rare because the discomfort felt in the hand is considered to be tolerable. However, it needs to be seriously treated when drugs and injections are no longer effective on the pain or discomfort. However, it needs to be operated on quickly before significant deformities occur, making an operation impossible. The aim of the operation is to correctly realign the bones and thus to decrease pain. Fitting a prosthesis, due to osteoarthritis, is extremely rare.

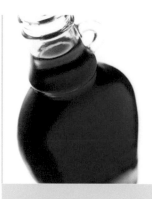

Vinegar of the four thieves

The reputation of plants was ambiguous for a long time. Thus a "witch" used digitalis both to poison her enemies and to treat heart disorders. When about to be burned at the stake, she traded her secret to save her life. Thus digitalis was introduced into our pharmacopoeia. In Toulouse, during a terrible plague epidemic which killed more than 50,000 between 1628 and 1631, four thieves were caught when they were fleecing the victims, revealing the secret that kept them free from contagion. After that, with no mercy whatsoever, they were hung. It was a balsamic vinegar which contained absinthe, rosemary sage and nutmeg among other things. It still appeared in the Codex 1884 as the term "vinegar of the 4 thieves".

MEDICINAL PLANTS

From Roman Gaul to the Middle Ages: the introduction of phytotherapy

Under the influence of a disciple of Hippocrates, the great Galen, a Greek-Roman doctor of the 2nd century B.C., the Romans also started to use plants. This explains why medicinal herbs, during the Roman Gaul period and in the Middles Ages, became in favor.

To treat arthritic ankylosis, the Romans relied on thermal springs which they developed intelligently, hot sand baths, like they still use in Sicily, including warm baths in the sea, the ancestors of our modern-day thalassotherapy.

Plants ranked high in their therapeutic arsenal. Rheumatism, which affected the lower classes who worked hard but also famous individuals like Cicero or the emperor Augustus, were also mainly treated with herbs belonging to the large family of Labiates: sage, thyme, wild thyme and rosemary. Galen wrote numerous formulas, long considered effective and was the creator of the "galenic" or science of medicines.

Certain plants were also used with malice to eliminate trouble-makers. The infamous "sorcerer's potions" contained digitalis, autumn crocus, belladonna and henbane. The evil Gilles de Rais, from near Nantes, used poppy seeds and jimsonweed to weaken his unfortunate victims so that he could better sexually abuse them before strangling them. Fortunately, these monsters which a miniscule minority. Plant medicine flourished in its true vocation which is to treat and relieve. Nature that helps humans in their suffering is good.

Hildegard's remedies

SSaint Hildegard admirably described that tumultuous period. This women, born to an aristocratic family, entered the Benedictine order at age fourteen. She became the abbess of one of the most beautiful Benedictine abbeys in Bavaria, the Rupertsberg abbey, near Bingen, was in turn a magnificent mystic and without doubt the first female doctor. And what a doctor! She inscribed her faith in sublime music which possessed lyrics and her science in remarkable treatises. She also wrote the four "Physica": before teaching Christ, you must heal the ill. She collected information from all her predecessors. She listened to all the traditional recipes. She studied hundreds of plants. After her, each monastery would have the courage to have its own botanical garden where medicinal herbs were grown to be put to use for the most humble..

Hildegard's joint treatments

Saint Hildegard introduced arnicato therapy, so useful for the joints, but also hawkweed, now known for its diuretic, uricolytic and bacteriostatic properties. Hildegard recommended baths, plasters and salves with badger fat. She also recommended, to relieve lombalgia,wearing a badger fur belt and massages with St. John's wort oil.

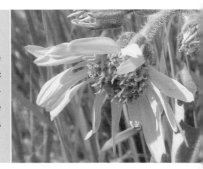

Paracelsus and the theory of signatures

With the Renaissance on the horizon, the shadow of Paracelsus appeared on the scene. And what a genius. Theophrastus Bombastus von Hohenheim, born in 1493 and died in 1541 at the age of 48, would revolutionize medicine.

A doctor, alchemist and Rosicrucian mystic, Paracelsus managing lots of work and difficult to decipher books, the Hermetic analogies which uniting the microcosm which is man, immersed in the plant and vegetable world, with the infinite macrocosm which is the universe, the same image of God.

As above, so below. Disease, death originating from divergence, an imbalance, an "antipathy" which breaks the sacred tie of cosmic "sympathy".

Provided that we know how to respect and complete them, the natural order of things, the beauty of divine creation are there to help us repair all the chaos caused by men. Disease is a major disorder. Nature provides the nearby remedy, available to the unfortunate sufferer. Minerals and plants containing all of the keys to health.

You just need to see them, to recognize them, by deciphering the « signs » offered to our senses. This is the "doctrine of the signatures".

Digitalis secret

The more the signature is secret and hidden away, the more the plant is active. Like alchemists, you need to know how to dig, burn, grind and distort to discover. Thus the petiole of the digitalis leaves when looked at from the side have the shape of a heart. So it is a remedy for heart disease. The magical appeal is great which opens the door to remarkable intuitions. Magic has its own lure, but it needs to be considered as an intuition which should lead to serious scientific research.

The similars

Each healing plant contains or bears the "signature" of the disease it cures. The stem of the horsetail is a miniature version of our spine. It is a remedy for demineralized, fragile and deformed spines.

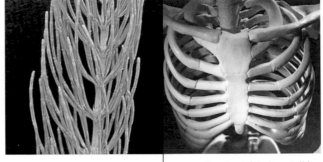

The stem of the horsetail is a miniature version of our skeleton.

Modern phytotherapy has confirmed horsetail's properties which are due to its high silica contents. The willow tilts towards the river. It is supposed to cure rheumatism which bends the body and is worsened by dampness. And even here, the discovery of salicylic acid has confirmed this. Greater celandine and golden seal secret a yellow sap. They treat jaundice or hepatitis. The euphrasia flower looks like our pupil. The plant treats eye problems, it is also called "eyebright". The doctrine of signatures was created as illustrated by Oswald Crollius and Robert Fludd. The last reincarnation of this doctrine by anthroposophists is without doubt the use of bamboo, like the horsetail, similar to our spine, for the treatment of spinal rheumatisms. The anthroposophist Rudolf Steiner also referred to the signature, for example in the analogies established between a tumor generated by mistletoe, Viscum album, on a tree and certain forms of neoplastic tumors. But here as well, a reliable scientific method needs to verify and confirm the intuitive phenomenon so that it can be considered by doctors who must remain individuals of science.

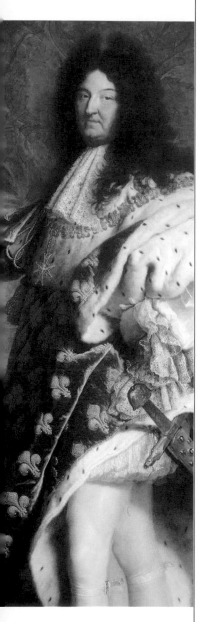

The age of scientific medicine

Starting in the 17th century with the introduction of new plants in Europe, medicine acquired analysis and evaluation tools, that still exist.

Louis XIV did much during this century to popularize plants. He introduced cinchona, named after a countess, to the kingdom. The powder of cinchona, brought by the Conquistadors of Peru, is useful for treating malaria. French doctors wanted nothing to do with it. The king imposed it.

In 1650, his ambassador to Lisbon, Nicot de Villemain, offered Marie de Médicis powdered tobacco brought by the Portuguese caravels, who liked it just as much as the Aztecs.

Cocoa was also introduced to the Court, then coffee given to the king by Soliman Aga, the Turkish ambassador. Later, Voltaire would drink more than twenty cups a day at the "la Procope" cafe in Paris.

Lastly, tea imported by the Dutch around 1666 arrived in Paris.

Knowledge becomes more refined

This scientific medicine, after plenty of false starts, was finally born. Paracelsus had spread the seeds. Alchemy generated chemistry, the plant signature and the discovery of the active ingredient. And finally Theriac arrived, the miracle salve that mixed everything aimed at healing everything. Thomas Sydenham dedicated himself to this at the end of 17th century with an in-death study on the analgesic benefits of opium. He invented the famous Laudanum which, before intoxicating Baudelaire, relieved a lot of pain.

At the origin of homeopathy, Samuel Hahnemann with the help of his pharmacist friend Franz Hartman defined the picking conditions for plants, the parts to use, their use in the form of a mother tincture prepared from fresh plants and maceration, dilution and potentization techniques.

Homeopathy: first plants

In 1810 Hahnemann published his extraordinary "The Organon of the Healing Art". It describes homeopathy which he invented and ways for scientifically experimenting with medications on humans thanks to the game of similars. By dilution and potentization, he extracted from plants - plant medications are more numerous in homeopathic pharmacopoeia – a remarkable energy for therapeutic activity. Thus Rhus toxicodendron, poison ivy; Bryonia doica, bryony; Rhododendron, rhododendron and; Phytolacca, American pokeweed would be great homeopath remedies for rheumatisms.

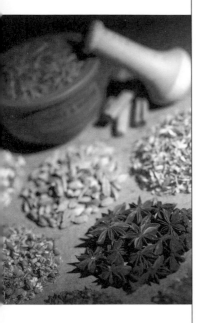

Looking for active ingredients

Starting from the 19th century considerable effort was made to identify and isolate the active ingredients contained in plants and obtain the pure state.

In 1806, morphine was extracted from opium. After having isolated emetine from ipecac (1817) and strychnine from nux vomica (1818), the pharmacists Pierre-Joseph Pelletier and Joseph-Bienaimé Caventou extracted quinine from cinchona in 1820, giving the world a weapon against the blight of malaria (periodic fever where the carrier is a mosquito). Claude-Adolphe Nativelle isolated digitalis from digitalin which he obtained in a crystallized state (1869).

Then came the great period of alkaloid extraction, of drugs called "heroic": atropine from belladonna, colchicine from colchicum, hyoscyamine, aconitine and cocaine among others.

Influenced by a slightly reductionist scientific spirit, the use of medicinal plants gradually fell out of use in favor of the isolated active ingredient. The idea was to obtain a clearer, faster and better targeted action. The chemical industry got involved, extracting, crystallizing and inven-

Freud: from cocaine to psychoanalysis

Before discovering psychoanalysis, Freud distinguished himself by testing cocaine extracted from the coca leaf as an eye analgesia, unwittingly turning one of his best friends into a cocaine addict.

ting by synthesis increasingly active derivatives, but also increasingly toxic. Paul Erlich starting with salicylic acid isolated from willow bark synthesized acetylsalicylic acid by acetylation. His example would be followed by numerous researchers.

The revival of phytotherapy

It wouldn't be until the 20th century when doctors, disenchanted with the results of these remedies, returned to the use of whole plants, well-known in popular medicine. The work of the French phytotherapy school, with first and foremost the wonderful Dr Henri Leclerc, but also Dr François Decaux de Vittel, and those conducted with Dr Claude Bergeret for the Société médicale de biothérapie relaunched the use of "natural" plants in medicine. University courses were set up including the departments at Lille, Bobigny and Besançon.

This phenomenon expressed the desire of patients who wanted to be treated effectively with non-aggressive, natural methods, supporting the forces of nature. This explains the remarkable current development of plant medicine. The discovery of medication forms easy to find in a drugstore, easy to absorb, with reliable storage and activity, the publication of specialized journals, appearance of adapted laws explains this rise. A renewal of the prescription with the arrival of aromatherapy of Dr Jean Valnet, gemmotherapy from us and Pol Henry and Bach flowers undeniably broaden the current field of phytotherapy.

Medicine through plants has an admirable, high-ranking future. Even if it can't treat everything, it can treat a lot.

At the origins of phytotherapy

Two modest French doctors fought in the 19th century to resurrect the use of medicinal plants. François-Joseph Cazin, a country doctor in Artésis, published a lengthy practical and critical treatise in 1847 on medicinal plants.

Dr Auguste Soins christened plant medicine in 1865 with the name "Phytotherapy", from the Greek phuton, "plant". This name has remained. He studied alkekengi or bladder cherry in urinary problems of prostate adenoma.

IN WHAT FORM ARE PLANTS USED?

Medicinal plants can be used both naturally or after pharmaceutical treatment in the form of various galenic preparation.

Plants used naturally

These are the traditional herb teas, well-loved by our grandmothers. They use only an isolated plant: meadowsweet herb tea, harpagophytum herb tea, solidago herb tea,

or a mixture of plants whose actions supported each other. Herb teas are prepared starting with different active parts of the plant, leaves, flowers or buds, roots or the whole plant. Both fresh and dry plants can be processed.

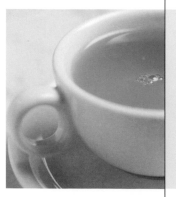

The marvelous pectoral herb tea

In the past there were also marvelous mixtures whose benefits were well known, for example the "pectoral herb tea", with great mullein, catsfoot and marshmallow among others, mixed with tussilago farfara, mallow, poppy and violet, a real summer bouquet blossoming deep in the country. It still appeared in the 1974 national formulary and has antitussive benefits, i.e. it makes it possible to expectorate and clean out clogged lungs.

There are two common herb tea preparation processes

- **The herb tea** is prepared by pouring a certain quantity of boiling water over the medicinal plant parts.
It is left to steep for 5 to 10 minutes. It is then filtered or strained. This is the traditional preparation process, for example for tea. In addition, the Germans and English call all herb teas "tea" and not just those made from Thea sinensis. They also have lime-blossom tea, mint tea, verbena tea, etc. The herb tea is reserved for the fragile parts of the flowers or leaves. Generally a teaspoon of pulverized dry plant is used for a cup of water, Since the active ingredients and flavors are volatile, the tea must be drunk quickly. You can also prepare meadowsweet, horsetail and heather tea to help your rheumatisms.

- **The brew** is prepared by emerging the plants in water which is brought to a boil un a closed container. It is left to boil for a bit with some reduction of the liquid. Obviously, the procedure makes it possible to extract more of the active substances and obtain more active concentrations which can be dangerous. It is reserved for plant parts which are hard to penetrate: roots, barks and seeds where the herb tea would extract little of the active ingredients. Thus you will prepare a pleasant white willow herb tea, effective against your pain by boiling 5 g of Salix alba branch bark per quart of water for 5 minutes.

An herb tea for rheumatisms

Herb tea is the most commonly used. Here is an excellent herb tea for rheumatisms, its formula is as follows: ash (leaves): 50 g, birch (leaves): 50 g, meadowsweet (buds): 50 g, anise (seeds): 50 g, red vine (leaves): 50 g, to mix.
1 teaspoon of this mixture in a mug of boiling water, let steep for 10 minutes. Effective and pleasant it should be drunk with moderation in the evening after dinner.

Galenic preparations of plants

Obviously, you can pick the plants to use yourself. But you need to be careful, you have to have precise botanical knowledge to start this endeavor and be able to tell the plants apart. This is the reason for the interest in looking for galenic preparations in the drugstore.

Medicinal plants are a bit like champignons. The toxic is side by side with the advantages. Every year you hear about intoxication from poisonous plants absent-mindedly picked by incompetent people unaware of the danger. Children are often victims of belladonna berries whose tempting appearance of small flat cherries makes them greedy. However, belladonna is a powerful poison.

So it is better to go to a drugstore with a good phyto-therapy section and to get single or mixed herb teas necessary for your rheumatisms and health.

There they have medications which need to be carefully composed, dosed at medicinal weights in compliance with preparation and storage rules. These preparations can only be used and delivered by specialist pharmacists.

The most common forms are gel capsules, extracts, alcoholatures, homeopathic tinctures, glycerin macerations and essential oils.

Gel capsules

These are prepared from pulverized plants whose nature, quality and active ingredient contents have been phar-macologically tested by serious, licensed pharmaceutical laboratories. The plant powders can be obtained by simple drying, pulverization and sifting, or by nebulization.

Nebulization is a technique used to obtain a finely pulverized dry extract from a very fast drying process which protects the properties of the plant. It entails drying a real spray of liquid particles emitted by an atomizer, a disk rotating at 50,000 turns per minute, inside a drying chamber crossed by very hot air. In a fraction of a second, the dried particles fall into very fine powder to be recovered and packaged.

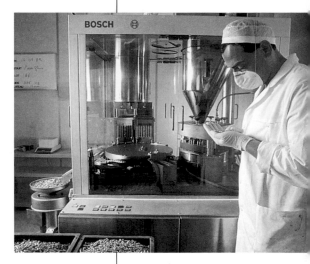

It is important to note that to avoid all "mad cow" problems the gel capsules are now made from plants.

Extracts

The pulverized plant is processed with water (aqueous extract) or alcohol (alcoholic extract). And a solution is obtained which evaporates until the desired concentration is reached. There are fluid extracts, with a low concentration, soft extracts, concentrated to a consistency of a loose paste and dry extracts which are very concentrated to pulverize..

The other Galenic preparations

Alcoholatures

These are obtained from the maceration of fresh plants in alcohol. Rich in enzymes, they do not last long since they ferment quickly. So they need to be used quickly..

Homeopathic mother tinctures

They are not close to traditional phytotherapy since they are homeopathic medications, the first degree of a range of dilution to be prescribed according to the law of Similars. But the similar justifiably makes it possible to emit a certain number of indications where, at ponderable doses, they will be useful to those who want to treat themselves with plants.

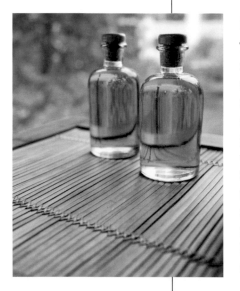

Plant mother tinctures (MT)

These are prepared according to very precise regulations defined by French pharmacopoeia and now by European pharmacopoeia. These mother tinctures of plant drugs are obtained by maceration of fresh plants, or more rarely, dried plants. They correspond to a tenth of their weight in dried drug, with the exception of Calendula MT (marigold tincture, greatly used for its cicatrizing properties), which corresponds to the twentieth. To prepare this mother tinctures, well-defined harvesting conditions have been established by the law. The plants which are used must be picked preferably in their natural habitat, which often excludes the use of cultiva-ted plants. After picking and identification of the plants by an expert pharmacist, the actual preparation of the mother tincture begins with alcoholic maceration for 3 weeks. There are almost 2000 different MT, this explains the scale and prescription flexibility of this range.

Glycerin macerations

These preparations are created by maceration to 1:20 in a mixture of water-alcohol-glycerin. They are used for buds and other plant tissues of an embryonic nature. They are the basis of a special therapeutic method, gemmotherapy whose rheumatology indications are completely remarkable.

Essential oils

Used in aromatherapy, these are usually obtained through distillation with water but also by expression and more rarely by incision for camphor of Borneo. The manufacturing technique quality for these essential oils is fundaments. The natural oils have an activity which is greatly superior to synthetic oils. In rheumatology the essential oils of juniper, birch and savory are used frequently among others, after dilution and in local massages, for example. But they can be toxic if the doses are too high. It is necessary to strictly follow the recom-mended dosages and not give them to children or pregnant women.

HARPAGOPHYTUM, THE "DEVIL'S CLAW"

Harpagophytum due to its analgesic and anti-inflammatory properties on joint pain, represents the most important innovation in recent years, in rheumatic medicine with plants.

An African plant

Harpagophytum procumbens a member of the Pedaliaceae botanical family has been christened the "Devil's Claw", a frightening name which does not imply any toxicity.

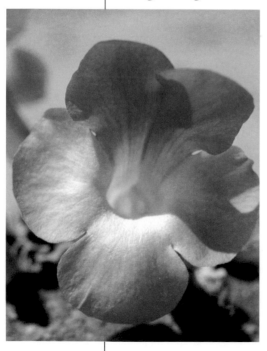

The plant comes from southwest Africa. It is mainly found in Namibia, whose capital Windhoek, has also given it the name of Windhoek root. It can also be found in Botswana and South Africa in the province of Cape and the Transvaal. It is picked in the sandy desert of Kalahari, a vast arid sandy plain extending at 3900 feet in altitude between the Zambezi and Orange rivers. In this savannah where the main vegetation is composed of rare prickly bushy undergrowth, the harpagophytum blossoms delicately.

Harpagophytum blooms in thin corolla, in the shape of blooming tubes whose pale crimson purple coloring shimmers in the vast sun of the desert. In these arid expanses, there is nothing prettier nor more surprising than this ode of hope facing the scorching sun.

But this beauty reveals a tragic trap in the fruits which generate these poetic flowers. They are actually hard capsules like wood studded with thorns and sharp hooks which energetically cling to anything they come into contact with, which is where the name harpago "I cling" comes from, actually the Greek harpaghos for the grappling iron, found in the etymology of words like "harpoon" or even "harpagon", the character of Molière who inspired Uncle Scrooge.

This "Devil's Claw" is thus capable of painfully injuring the paws and hooves of animals but also the bare feet of unfortunate Zulus running in the savannah to track game. The trapped animal furiously struggles to free itself from these deadly needles whose removal for humans is as tough as that of the the spines of an urchin you may encounter on the pretty Mediterranean.

Very early on, African shamans learned how to use a brew of its strangely shaped root to treat different complaints: constipation, migraines and hives. The action against joint and spine, osteoarthritis and arthritis pain was discovered by German botanical missions and confirmed by western clinical medicine.

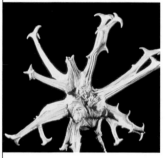

The thorn studded fruit

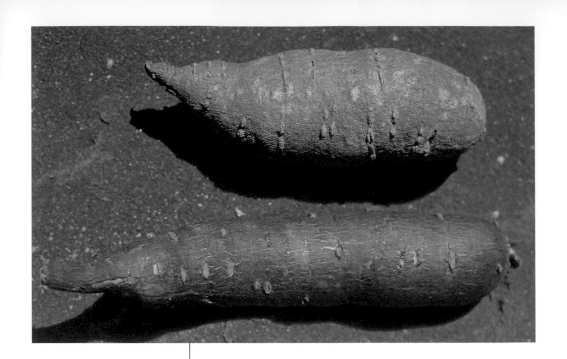

Everything is in the root

Harpagophytum is a small perennial herbaceous plant with opposing leaves whose root is made of an axis vertically piercing the soil up to 3 feet in depth to search for the water necessary for its growth. Secondary roots sprout from this main root bearing large protuberances which can weigh up to 500 grams. This is their volume. These are the tubers which constitute the medicinal part of the drug.

The harpagophytum tubers, the only medicinal part containing:

- dwaxes and fatty acids;
- sugars and sugar by-products;
- flavonoids, colored pigments;
- phytosteroids, phenols, all substances frequently found in the plant kingdom but whose presence strengthens and enhances the therapeutic benefits of the active ingredients.

These active ingredients have been identified as being iridoids, chemical substances with a highly original structure and remarkable anti-inflammatory properties.

The most important of these iridoids is harpagoside, glucoside which under the action of different ferments splits into very weak harpagogenin and sugars. Then comes harpagide, procumboside and procumbide.

The dry root of harpagophytum contains 0.5 to 3% iridoids whose presence explains the therapeutic activity of the drug but whose extreme weakness requires very scrupulous precautions when picking and storing the plant.

All harpagophytums on the market do not have the same value and you need to be very careful and ask for the pharmaceutical label.

A well-guarded secret

From 1902 to 1908 the German army had to face a revolt of local tribes, the Hottentots, in Namibia, a revolt which was put down in blood. A soldier named Hubertus Mehnert noticed that the shamans used decoctions of a root to heal injured Hottentot warriors and this remedy seemed very effective. Despite the efforts of local healers to keep the Germans from identifying the miraculous plant the Germans finally figured it out. In 1904, the first harpagophytum samples left the African soil to be studied in Germany. You know the rest.

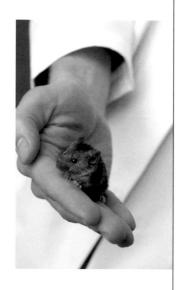

Proven anti-inflammatory properties

The harpagophytum iridoids are the best against painful inflammation of joints as shown by pharmacological studies.

The aqueous extract of harpagophytum inhibits the inflammatory swelling of rat paw caused by injection of formalin with decrease in the production of orosoniucoids, markers of inflammatory states as well as the edema resulting from injection of croton oil in rat and guinea pig.

Moreover, the anti-inflammatory activity tested on guinea pig is comparable to that of nonsteroidal anti-inflammatory drugs (NSAIDs), which is remarkable in itself. It is necessary to mention three recent drug studies which are particularly interesting, objectifying the anti-inflammatory and analgesic properties of Devil's Claw. Croton oil, a particularly caustic substance, is injected into rat paw. The result is the production of what is called an inflammatory granuloma, i.e. a sort of very painful sterile abscess which greatly swells the affected limb. And, the previous injection in the rat peritoneum of a harpagophytum extract for 12 days or even more simply administration by mouth, gives an identical result as that obtained with phenylbutazone, one of the most powerful anti-inflammatory drugs known, used in the past to neutralize major arthritis but practically abandoned at present due to its toxicity on the blood and white blood cells (Eichler and Koch, 1970).

Harpagophytum also acts on pain

In 1992, experiments demonstrated the analgesic effects of harpagophytum, all the more effective when the administered dose increases (Lanhers and Fleurentin, 1992). This is what is called a "dose-dependant effect". The test used the reaction to pain of different batches of mice after administration of harpagophytum extracts in the peritoneum (abdominal internal membrane). Reference was made to standardized scales to allow a quantitative approach to pain phenomenon. An analgesic effect was observed equal to:

- 47 % for a 100 mg dose of harpagophytum per kg;
- 78 % for a 400 mg/kg dose.

At a dose of 200 mg/kg a 53% analgesic protector effect was obtained which is equal to the protector effect (59 %) obtained with 68 mg of aspirin per kg. This result is remarkable, since in relation to a 60 kg man it represents 4 g of aspirin. In terms of the pure ingredient of harpagoside, it protects 42% for a minimum dose of 10 mg/kg. These are exciting figures.

Safe and effective

The anti-inflammatory action was studied in rats receiving an intramuscularly injection of adriamycin, an irritating and aggressive substance. The protector doses of orally administered harpagophytum were 37 mg/kg, 370 mg/kg and 3 700 mg/kg (Jadot and Lecomte, 1992). The obtained results show that from the weakest dose, our plant has a significant anti-inflammatory protector action. For very high doses (37 mg/kg, 3 700 mg/kg) i.e. 10 to 100 times the recommended doses in human treatment, an analgesia saturation is reached which is also at a maximum without detecting any toxic effect. This experiment demonstrated both the effectiveness and harmlessness of harpagophytum, the appropriate dose to use is around 37 mg/kg.

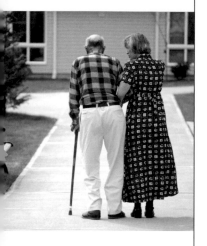

Harpagophytum relieves the joints

Numerous, rigorous studies have demonstrated the anti-rheumatic action of harpagophytum.

It was one of the first clinical studies conducted on a vast scale. Schmidt tested the effectiveness of harpagophytum on 100 rheumatic patients as a supplement to classical anti-inflammatory treatment (Schmidt, 1972). These were particularly severe rheumatisms, for example rheumatoid arthritis. The medication was administered by local injections on each side of the affected joints. This manner of administration has been totally abandoned because taking it by mouth is just as effective and much less restrictive. An improvement in the condition of these patients was obtained in 80% of the cases. In 60% of them, the pain disappeared totally and recovery of the joint was very satisfactory. In all cases, it was possible to decrease the doses of anti-inflammatory drugs by half. The eminent phytotherapy doctor Paul Belaiche, head of the phytotherapy department at Bobigny, tested an aqueous spray in gel capsules of harpagophytum titred at 2.5% harpagoside for a dosage of 3 g per days taken in three doses. 630 patients recruited from patients in the town were then tested. They suffered from different forms of osteoarthritis: osteoarthritis of hip, knee, osteoarthritis of the hands and feet, osteoarthritis of the spine, especially lumbar, all with a lot of pain. The improvement of the patients was very clear, naturally varying based on the severity of the rheumatism. After six months of treatment, there was only an 18.01% failure rate. In 21% of the cases, according to Belaiche, it was necessary to increase the dosage to 9 g per day, this did not cause any side effects.

The proof from clinical studies

Another work using nebulized gel capsules of harpagophytum was performed in a hospital on 50 osteoarthritis patients in a double blind test of the plant against (Guyaden, 1984). Each patient received in one or more sequences of 21 days in three daily doses nebulized harpagophytum, titred at 1.5% harpagoside, in order to absorb 36 mg of the active ingredient. Its effectiveness was measured on the different types of pain: at rest, active and passive mobilization, joint pressure, when walking, on nighttime pain causing wakening. The obtained scores were much higher with harpagophytum than the placebo: 72% of positive cases with harpagophytum, 54% with the placebo. Some digestion problems were recorded: minor nausea, gastralgia, diarrhea with one case of hives. Thus an effective and well tolerated treatment! One study tested Arkogélules®. The study demonstrated the effectiveness of these gel capsules on osteoarthritis joint pain and the lack of mobility resulting from ankylosis (Pinget and Lecomte, 1985). A rigorous double blind study was performed (Costa and Lecomte, 1992). The study was conducted on 89 osteoarthritis subjects divided into 2 groups. One received 2 g of harpagophytum extract titred at 3% of harpagoside per day in three doses. The other only received the placebo. A significant decrease in the intensity of joint pain was observed and an increase in mobility of the spine. Even the hip joint was better, which is a good result for patients with this type of osteoarthritis. No toxic or undesirable effect was observed.

How do you use harpagophytum?

Harpagophytum procumbens **commonly used in two forms easy to get in a drugstore. These are the ones you need to get and learn how to take.**

Harpagophytum is indicated for the treatment of all rheumatic pain, no matter what its location. It is used alone or as a supplement to traditional anti-rheumatic therapies. Harpagophytum has only one contraindication, but it is important: pregnancy because it can cause a premature delivery. Harpagophytum is also not recommended during nursing.

Harpagophytum exists in various forms:

• solid form, dry powder capsule or nebulized harpagophytum titered in harpagoside and in gel capsules generally with a dose of 400 mg. The daily dosage is 2 to 6 gel capsules per day, 3 gel capsules for maintenance;
• liquid form, a mother tincture, prepared according to the rules of homeopathic pharmacopoeia. The dosage is 80 drops in the morning and at night (1 measure) to take in a large glass of water. You start with a continuous treatment of 1 or 2 months based on the intensity of the pain phenomena. Then you take intermittent treatments of 20 days per month. It is always a good idea to take a break from treatment, for example 1 month out of 3.

A safe plant

This plant does not have any toxicity. The lethal dose of 50 determined on mice, which means that it kills 50% of the small rodents, an obligatory drug test for all medications on the market, is remarkably high: 1 g/kg for harpagoside; 3,2 g/kg for harpagide. The powder of the root does not give any toxic effect on rat at the very high dose of 3 g/kg! The absence of side effects and above all the good tolerance of the stomach, authorizes long-term treatments necessary in chronic rheumatisms.

The Max Tétau study (2001)

A clinical test was conducted by Max Tétau on medical patients for different forms of osteoarthritis with harpagophytum MT. 50 patients were selected for each form of rheumatism. Dosage: 80 drops in the morning and at night for a duration of 2 months, a break for 1 months and 2 months again. Here are the results:

	TB	B	AB	0
Cervical	55 %	15 %	20 %	10 %
Lumbar	60 %	10 %	25 %	5 %
Hip	45 %	15 %	30 %	10 %
Knee	58 %	12 %	15 %	15 %
Shoulder	54 %	16 %	12 %	18 %
Osteoarthritis: toes, fingers	53 %	17 %	20 %	10 %

Legend:
TB: disappearance of the pain and ankylosis. Elimination of all painkillers.
B: significant improvement. Acetaminophen, traditional painkiller remains necessary at times.
AB: moderate but real improvement. Taking painkillers remains frequent.
0 : no improvement. Traditional treatment needs to be maintained. Thus failure.

An example of treatment

Ms. L, 52 years old, secretary-bookkeeper comes for consultation for persistent, disabling neck pain. Her work on a computer does not help things. She complains of shooting pain at the level of the nape, aggravated by the slightest movement of her head, going down her left arm with numbness in the last three fingers of the hand. Rotation of her head is particularly painful. At night Ms. L had to sleep with her neck blocked by a firm bolster. An x-ray revealed unquestionable severe signs of osteoarthritis mainly at the 5th, 6th and 7th cervical vertebrae. Since Ms. L had been treated for hiatus hernia and gastric reflux by a proton pump inhibitor, she could not be given corticosteriods, NSAIDs, or even simple aspirin. Only acetaminophen was authorized. So I prescribed harpagophytum powder in 2 gel capsules of 400 mg morning, noon and night, associated with wearing a flexible cervical collar (a neck brace) for three days both day and night, and the other three days only during the daytime. Ms. L returned three weeks later, she was happy to report an improvement in her condition. Her nape was much more flexible and much, much less painful. The numbness in her fingers had disappeared. We advised Ms. L to continue the treatment for a month but with 2 gel capsules morning and night. And since then everything has been fine.

TEN PLANTS FOR RELIEVING PAIN

There are more than 21,000 plants which are attributed with various medicinal properties. Our selection is targeted to those plants capable of acting directly or indirectly on your suffering joints without the risk of poisoning you.

We have gathered some "medicinal herbs" with pain-killing properties able to neutralize pain, which can lower your uric acid and stimulate your kidneys, and cicatrize joint cartilage. These are plants growing in the surrounding countryside. You just have to bend over to pick them, as long as you know them. So here are the 10 plants for your joint happiness, the first is fennel.

Fennel
(*Foeniculum vulgare*, *Umbelliferae* family)

Fennel, in abundant supply along country paths, is a wonderful plant.

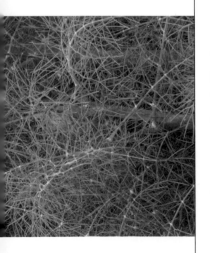

The Ancients had made this herb, very widespread around the Mediterranean, into a symbol of the Sun God. They burned this plant during sacrifices they offered to the gods and the fragrant fennel fumes contributed to their sacred exhilaration while teasing the nostrils of the gods. Dioscorides recommended it "to those who can only piss drop by drop."

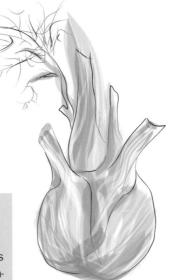

Fennel a jack of all trades

Fennel stimulates digestion. An herb tea made with fennel seeds drunk warm after a heavy meal calms the heartburn of an irritated stomach, a heavy liver and accelerates digestion. It is also used to treat excess weight and dissolves the accumulation of cellulite. It reduces edemas.

Fennel includes many wild varieties. One species is cultivated, it has a very pleasant taste and the fleshy base at the bottom of the stocks is eaten. The plant is highly aromatic. It releases a fresh fragrance due to an essence rich in anethol which gives it its characteristic

aniseed flavor. Fennel has two therapeutic properties which primarily interest us here.

It quickly relieves joint pains, whether it is eaten or used topically. Poultices of fresh fennel stalks and leaves applied to a painful joint are a rejuvenating experience for osteoarthritis sufferers. It is also an interesting diuretic and promotes the elimination of water, urea and uric acid all toxic substances which devastate the rheumatic.

Fennel treatments in spring and fall, very damp seasons when rheumatism flourishes, will be particularly welcome. You can also take it in summer to lose weight, and acquire a good figure for the beach.

DOSAGE

2 gel capsules morning and night;
20 days per month;
2 to 3 months
or *Foeniculum* tincture,
80 drops at lunch
and dinner.

A recipe for the holidays

The roots of asparagus, holly, apium, parsley and fennel are used to make the traditional "five root syrup", an old diuretic and purifying medication with a caramel flavor. Some drugstores still make it: 1 to 2 soup spoons a day in a large glass of water, for 1 or 2 weeks, after the holiday season.

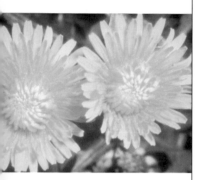

Dandelion

(*Taraxacum dens leonis*, *Compositae* family)

"Suck dandelions from the roots" is not always a bad sign.

One of my 80 year old patients astonished me with his sprightliness. Slim and slender, this brilliant but needy eighty year old still wandered around Paris on a doddery scooter to sell insurance policies necessary for his subsistence and that of a completely recent family since this deserving old man was a "relatively" young bridegroom with a 12 year old girl to raise.

The flexibility of this man was remarkable. He was unaware of his joints, and had never heard anyone talk about them. His secret: an herb tea of dandelion root every night.

He picked it himself in fall or February and let it dry gently in the oven of his range to ensure his stock for a year. The herb tea is bitter but the result was there. This alert man makes it by steeping 20 g of dried roots with a quart of water. "Sucking dandelions from the roots" is thus not always a bad sign since my patient happily lived past age 95 in astonishing conditions and died after a fall when he fractured his femur. It was around 1546 when Bock, a German doctor, reported the medicinal properties of dandelion for the first time. But it was one of his fellow countrymen, an apothecary with the sumptuous name of Tabernaemontus, who made it a real panacea for its highly diuretic properties. The dandelion is actually a diuretic, it greatly improves the elimination of water and uric acid. But it is also a marvelous detoxifying agent and liver tonic due to the sterols and bitter lactones and cholagogues it contains.

DOSAGE
2 powder gel capsules at lunch and dinner, 15 days per month or Taraxacum MT, 50 to 100 drops a day.

Proof of its purifying action, it will lower your blood cholesterol and triglycerides with repeated treatments. It has a general action on your body which works on the joints resulting in more flexibility and less pain. I suggest you eat its leaves, primarily those picked in the spring, with salads dressed with olive oil and lemon juice. From a medical viewpoint, you can get back into shape with a dandelion treatment very beneficial for you and which was very popular during the past century.

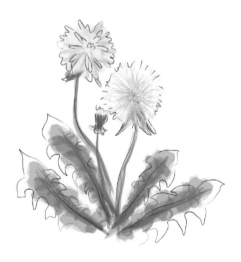

The postal worker and dandelion

So Mr. Louis D., age 50, a postman, had blood tests done in January, which revealed 3 g of cholesterol and 100 mg of uric acid. After 3 months of treatment with dandelion, his cholesterol lowered to 2.40 g and his uric acid to 70 mg.

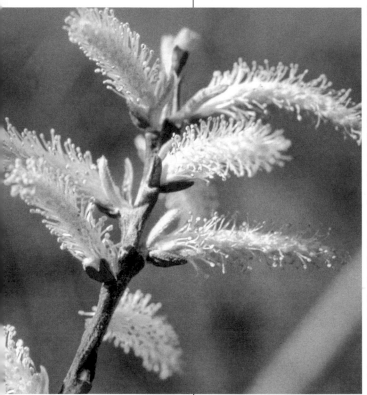

White willow

(*Salix alba*, , family of *sali-caceae*)

In the 17th century Mattioli reported the effectiveness of the leaves in an enema against insomnia. But starting in the 16th century it was used to treat rheumatic pain.

The theory of the signatures which in the past attributed medicinal properties to plants based on their shape and where they grew, considered that willows, living harmoniously with their "feet" in the water, should treat chills, fever, the flu and joint pain. It was once called, "the tree for all aches".

The white willow, still called the white osier, is a tree which grows in much of the northern hemisphere. More than two hundred species of Salix exist possessing adaptation qualities to very cold climates and altitudes which are completely astonishing. But more than anything else it is a tree which loves water. Salix alba grows in Europe on river banks and in humid forests. It is the bark which is medicinal. Doctors in Antiquity attached great importance to it. Struck by its effectiveness, Erlich analyzed the

DOSAGE
1 powder gel capsules at breakfast, lunch and dinner *Salix* tincture, 40 to 50 drops a day. Herb tea: boil 5 g of branch bark per quart of water.

leaves and bark and extracted significant quantities of salicylic acid from a heteroside, salicin where this acid is combined with a sugar. It is starting from this salicylic acid that the first synthesis of aspirin would be created, acetylsalicylic acid, whose analgesic action has relieved millions of human beings around the world. The bark of the white willow is also suited for rheumatics, whose stomach is often attacked by analgesics and anti-inflammatory drugs, since it is eupeptic, thus soothing for the gastric mucous membrane thanks to its tannins. Willow is prescribed for hyperchlorhydric dyspepsia, 20 to 50 drops a day.

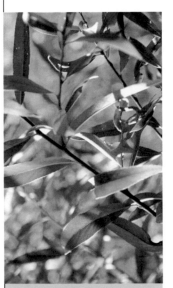

For "excessive" women

The fluid extract of catkins of white willow are recommended for women who suffer from rheumatisms but also from an "excessive temperament" if if such excessiveness is pathological and not a pleasure for her and her partner.

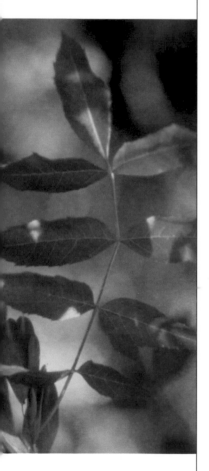

Ash

(*Fraxinus excelsior*, family of *Oleaceae*)

Diuretic, anti-rheumatic and laxative, the leaves of the ash have the reputation of slowing aging.

The ash is a very pretty tree with its slender trunk, slightly grayish bark and ethereal foliage. It belongs to a highly evolved group of plants, without doubt one of the most recent to appear on our planet. Its leaves, formed of seven to fifteen leaflets, are medicinal. They need to be picked young, in June, still covered with their sugary, sticky coating. Rich in tannins, sugars, resins, Vitamin C, minerals, especially zinc, they contain glucosides and malic acid. Study of its chemical composition reveals the presence of a flavonoid, rutin, with anti-inflammatory properties. The diuretic activity is due to mannitol and potassium salts present in the leave which make it possible to stimulate the body's elimination functions. Ash leaves, anti-inflammatory and diuretic, are thus indicated for treating rheumatisms, osteoarthritis, gout as well as water retention problems and edema. We now know that mannitol is captures free radicals and that polyphenols are antioxidants. These

Frenette

A long time ago, our fellow countrymen drank what was called frenette, a slightly acid beverage obtained by fermenting fresh ash leaves in sugary water. They considered it healthy and refreshing. It fought the the stiffness that they earned from hard work in the fields.

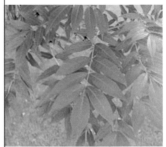

properties make it possible to use these substances as tissue protectors of joints, stopping their aging. Dr.Henri Leclerc was very interested in the anti-aging benefits of ash. By macerating the leaves in a sugar syrup, he prepared an elixir whose merits he boasted about to his aged patients stunned by rheumatism. He also drank it and remained sharp to a ripe old age.

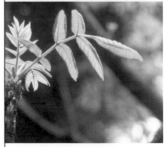

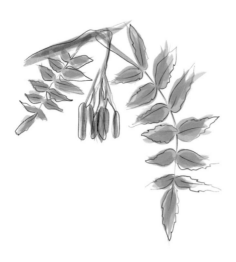

DOSAGE

2 gel capsules at lunch, 2 at dinner, 20 days per month; *Fraxinus* tincture: 50 drops, 1 to 2 times a day. Herb tea: 15 g of leaves per quart, one cup after dinner. This ash treatment is diuretic, revitalizing and relaxing.

Meadowsweet

(*Spires ulmaria*, , family of *Rosaceae*)

The presence in the fresh plant of different salicyles, in particular monotropitoside a generator of alkaline salicylates and methyl, gives it clear anti-rheumatic properties.

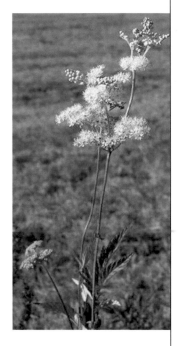

Meadowsweet is a pretty herbaceous plant which loves moist places, on the edges of steams, in water-filled prairies, on the edges of marshes. Its haughty bearing, pretty ivory white tuft, make it easy to recognize. Its fragrance is pleasant and subtle and attracts pollen-gathering bees.

Already well-known by Medieval botanists, Albertus Magnus and Saint Hildegard of Binden, its main medicinal properties came to light during the Renaissance and were later confirmed in the 19th century. The healthy action of the plant is due to the presence, in the flowery tops, of flavonoids and above all salicyle derivatives, precursors of the most widespread medicine in the world: aspirin.

These products give meadowsweet an anti-inflammatory and analgesic action used for treating painful joints (rheumatisms and osteoarthritis).

Its effects are gentle and progressive and perfectly well-tolerated.

A study conducted in 1989 against a placebo showed that meadowsweet, in association with blackcurrant, constitutes an effective basic treatment for chronic rheumatic disease.

DOSAGE
2 gel capsules at lunch, 2 at dinner *Spires* MT: 50 to 100 drops a day
Herb tea: 20 g of the dried tops to steep for 5 minutes. in a quart of water, never let it boil or it will destroy the salicylates.

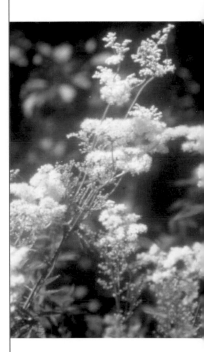

It makes it possible to significantly decrease the need for traditional analgesics and anti-inflammatory drugs which are aggressive for the body in the long term, mainly causing important side effects for the digestion system.

The plant also dilates the veins, tones the heart and and accelerates diuresis. Its numerous properties justify its indication in weight loss treatments: it improves the kidneys' elimination of water, the reabsorption of painful edemas and can combat cellulite and obesity.

It perfectly enhances the action of harpagophytum.

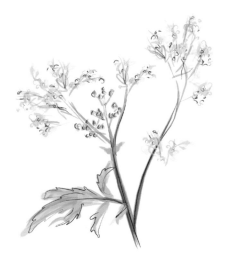

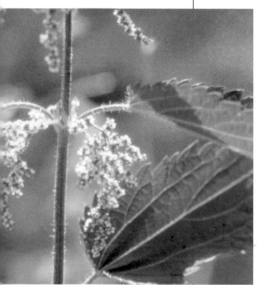

Nettle

(*Urtica dioica*, , family of *Urticaceae*)

Theophrastus, Dioscorides and Pliny mentioned it for relaxing stiff joints, Paracelsus attributed it with the greatest benefits: "You will respect the diabolic nettle. She will bring you well-being." Already something bad to get well!

The great forbidding nettle shoots its stinging hairs across all of temperate Europe. Who hasn't been stung by nettles? The substance responsible for the fierce burning which occurs on contact is complex.

The sting of the nettle releases chemical mediators in the skin identical to those responsible for allergic reactions. These include histamine, acetylcholine and formic acid. This burning sap is contained in the hollow hairs located on the leaf petioles. Their fragile tips enter the skin and release their poison. There is also a much more aggressive nettle, the dwarf nettle or Urtica urens. It is the smallest in size but all of its foliage is covered with stinging hairs. The aerial part of the nettle contains numerous active ingredients: vitamins of the B group, A, C, E, minerals such as magnesium, iron or silica and trace elements (copper, zinc, etc.).

It is its richness in silica, zinc but also vitamins which makes it very useful for treating brittle nails and split ends.

DOSAGE
2 gel capsules morning and night (gel capsules of the root or pulverized leaves)
Urtica dioica MT:
50 to 100 drops a day.
Herb tea: 1 teaspoon of dry leaves for 1 cup of water.
Salve, with the following formula: *Urtica urens* MT 10 g, non-greasy transcutaneous excipient as needed 50 g massage very gently.

It is a good remineralizer which, thanks to the iron and folic acid, can be recommended for treating worn cartilage in people who suffer from osteoarthritis or rheumatisms, particularly during menopause. Lastly, nettle is known for its tonic and anti-asthenic properties and thanks to its iron content it is a good supplement for pregnant women. I remember having quickly relieved a painful shoulder periarthritis of a fanatic golfer with this salve. It had been resistant to the strongest traditional anti-inflammatory drugs. And plus a few young shoots of this small nettle thrown into a good vegetable soup add an excellent flavor and some benefits.

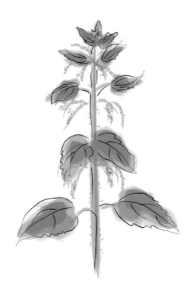

A barbaric treatment

Nettle was used in herb teas prepared from fresh leaves. Rheumatics were also advised to roll around in nettle bushes or to beat themselves with freshly picked stalks. The resulting revulsion relieved joint pain. They also wove the stalks to make coarse belts, or even tunics, whose stinging improved lumbar and back pain. All of this now seems archaic, barbaric and a bit sadistic.

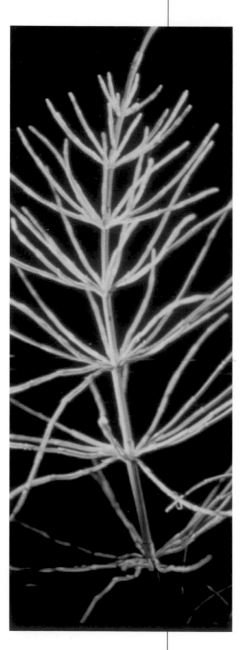

Horsetail

(Equisetum arvense, , family of Equiseta-ceae)

With this plant it is possible to fight demineralization, in particular the tragic osteoporosis which affects women after menopause.

LIn terms of botanical ecology, the horsetail is a very ancient plant which is mainly picked on sandy land. It is the heir of the great ferns of the Ice Age. Like ferns, it does not bloom and so it does not produce seeds. Reproduction is ensured by spores collected in spikes at the end of certain stems, spores containing an elastic tissue which lets them propel themselves by leaping like a flea or kangaroo, which ensure the broad dispersion of this very common plant.

The horsetail has two types of stem. The first is reddish, without chlorophyll, it sprouts at the beginning of spring and bears the fertile spike. When fertilization is complete, they wilt and tall green stems appear which are grooved and very bushy, similar to a fox tail. Only these sterile stems are medicinal and they should be picked in the summer.

This unusual rhythm of life has attracted a lot of attention. In addition, the « signature » of the stem, which somewhat resembles the spine, indicates a possible action on it. The discovery of horsetail's extraordinary mineral richness, particularly in silicon, has made it possible to better understand the action mechanisms of this plant. It stimulates the synthesis of collagen contained in the bone and connective tissues, which improves cartilage reformation during joint diseases. Subjects suffering from joint or rheumatism problems very much benefit from it with an improvement in their mobility. Silica also improves the mending of fractures by promoting the formation of bone callus. Its composition significantly improves the flexibility of tendons and helps to protect them during sustained sports. Silicon deficiencies are frequent and increase with age. This is the reason for the interest in regular treatments with horsetail to completely benefit from all its remineralizing effects. Horsetail possesses a diuretic effect which is the origin of its traditional use to improve elimination functions of the body and fight against water retention problems.

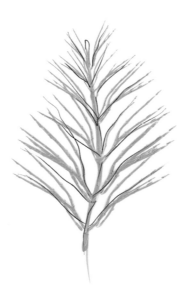

POSOLOGIE

2 to 3 gel capsules a day in intermittent treatments or a large cup of herb tea: 20 g per quart in an herb tea will help to strengthen a weakened skeleton. Equisetum MT: 50 to 100 drops a day to promote weight loss, and combating decalcification, in our friends experiencing menopause for 1 or 2 months.

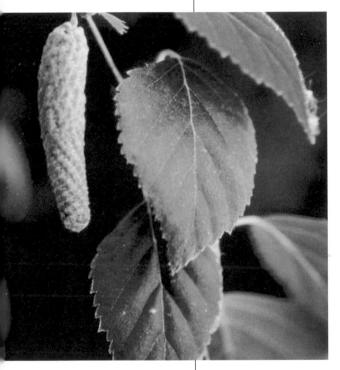

Birch

(*Betula alba var pubescens and verrucosa*,
family of *Betulaceae*)

It is the sap of the birch picked when it is fresh that we recommend for anti-osteoarthritis purposes.

The birch, also called tree of knowledge, is a magnificent tree. Its satiny bark with a silvery white color due to the presence of a wax, is the ornament of forests developed on sandy or siliceous land. It can be found all over Europe, except on the shores of the Mediterranean. In France, the Sologne birches are particularly pretty.

Their sugary sap is used to prepare a fermented elixir, rich in vitamins and trace elements. The Scandinavians considered it as a gift from the god Odin, the source of energy and youth (see the box).

The birch leaves contain flavonoids, namely hyperisode, with diuretic and depurative properties.

A birch treatment is useful for treating rheumatic pains and gout since it improves the elimination of chloride and uric acid.

DOSAGE
It is diluted at 10% and 50 to 100 drops are taken a day of birch sap. First Decimal (bottle of 125 ml).

It also prevents the formation of bladder stones. The birch is a draining diuretic plant: it is useful for treating water retention and edemas of the limbs frequently found in premenstrual syndrome.

We have pharmacologically studied the sap of the birch. We have isolated significant quantities of heterosides, salicin and betuloside from it able to release new salicylic acid, which is analgesic, anti-rheumatic and de-ankylosizing. It can be found in most drugstores.

The herb tea of birch leaves is less active.

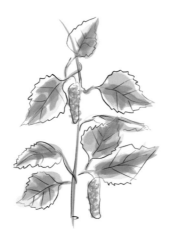

The tree with the sacred sap

In Nordic countries, the birch acquired sacred virtues and was part of a very ritualized folklore. During springtime in Lapland, Finland and Sweden, an entire ceremony requires the harvesting of birch sap. In a long procession, when this sap is tapped, the villagers go to the forest and cut the trees to collect the precious liquid flowing flowing from the cut and pouring in torrents in clear, light, crystalline and slightly frothy water.

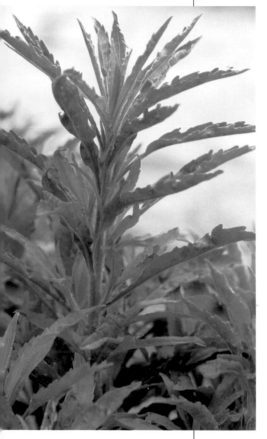

Horseweed

(*Erigeron canadense*, family of *Compositae*)

This is a remarkable uricolytic, an energetic joint anti-inflammatory. Dr. Henri Leclerc, the eminent phytotherapist introduced in around 1930 to pharmacies and Dr. Brel dedicated an important study to it.

This plant is originally from Canada. It appeared in Europe during the last century, undoubtedly brought by the bundles of some goods from America. After that it spread everywhere in Europe. It invaded our trails and our fallow lands. The plant contains an oil rich in acetylenic compounds similar to that of chamomile instead of limonene and choline.

Dr Henri Leclerc is his phytotherapy handbook included an exciting note: "A farmer came to see me who was condemned to lack of mobility and devastated by fierce suffering from a sacro-iliac arthritis. Since along with this problem he had the annoyance of seeing his crops invaded by the horseweed proliferating there, I enlisted him to use that bad herb to fight his painful and relentless affliction.

He had a strong decoction made (150 g in a quart of water) and he drank three glasses every morning. This treatment produced the most felicitous effect so that the patient who, before couldn't curse the indiscreet plant enough, started to consider it with an ambiguous expression, at times disapproving and grateful, like a roman-

DOSAGE
2 to 3 gel capsules a day
Erigeron MT 50
to 100 drops a day,
with a 1 to 2 month
treatment

tic poet would portray someone trying to stone a dog with succulent bones."

Study of the composition of this plant reveals the presence of flavones and tannins which give it both diuretic and anti-inflammatory properties. Thus it can be used successfully to treat rheumatisms and osteoarthritis, to relieve the pain of inflamed joints and to prevent gout. Its anti-rheumatic activity is reinforced by association with harpagophytum or blackcurrant.

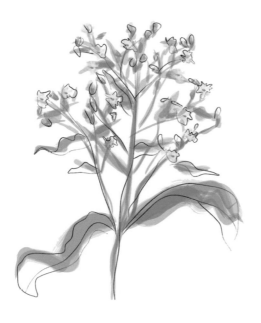

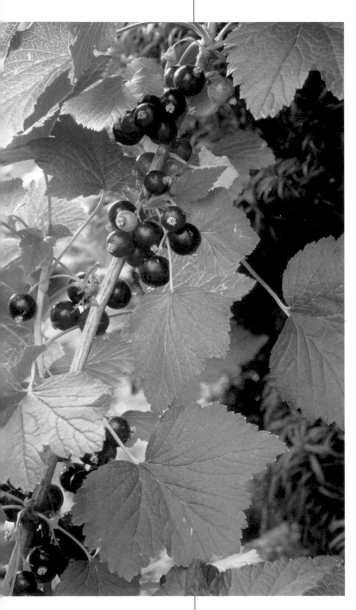

Blackcurrant

(*Ribes nigrum,* family of *Saxifragaceae*)

The blackcurrant lowers blood pressure, protects your veins and by slowing the inflammation process, it will fight your old pains.

Blackcurrant, a favorite of Rudolf Steiner's, the anthroposophist, is a remarkable remedy for rheumatic pain. The leaves and fruits are used in gel capsules or a mother tincture and its buds are the basis for gemmotherapy.

This small tree grows wild in northern and central Europe as well as in northern Asia. It is cultivated for its fruit and buds in several central European countries.

The blackcurrant leaves are rich in flavonoids (rutin and hyperoside), catechol tannins and C and P vitamins.

Thanks to their anti-rheumatic and anti-inflammatory properties, they act effectively in the case of acute or chronic painful joints, especially for osteoarthritis pain of the knee joint.

The blackcurrant leaves are also a strong diuretic promoting the elimination of waste (uric acid and toxins) by the body.

All of these properties make it possible to recommend blackcurrant leaves for the basic treatment of gout.

Here's to Caesar

According to tradition Julius Caesar when leading his armies to conquer Gaul, had the opportunity to taste a plate of blackcurrants served with a glass of good red Burgundy. He liked the fruit and asked for it at other meals. This French blackcurrant cure, considerably improved his joint flexibility, causing him to start the dual trend of wine and French blackcurrants in Rome, well before Chanoine invented kir.

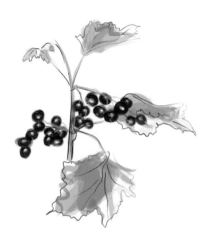

DOSAGE
Try this anti-rheumatic herb tea just as it has been handed down to us by Saint Hildegard and tradition: Dry meadowsweet and blackcurrant plants as needed for 200 g 1 soup spoon to steep for 10 minutes and a pint of boiling water. Filter. To be savored greedily, sweetened with rosemary honey, 1 cup after lunch and dinner.

GEMMOTHERAPY: THE STRENGTH OF BUDS

An original form of phytotherapy has developed in recent years. To treat different diseases it does not use the whole plant, but basically just the buds.

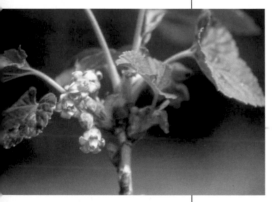

Blackcurrant buds

Promoters of the method with our friend Dr. Pol Henry of Brussels, we have called it gemmotherapy (from the Latin gemma, "bud"). Gemmotherapy uses glycerin macerations prepared from fresh plant buds. Due to their activity, only the first decimal is released.

For example, we use the buds of blackcurrant, hawthorn, birch and oak. Other plant tissues are added which are in the process of growing such as young shoots, rootlets and the inner part of stem bark. We recommend young rosemary or juniper shoots for the liver, corn rootlets are of interest for the heart, the inner stem bark of the lemon tree is an anticoagulant. These are all tissues which have maintained their embryonic capacities. As we have demonstrated with professor Netien from the faculty of Lyons, they are rich in active growth factors, auxins and and gibberellins.

These substances express the remarkable and precise activity of this real plant embryotherapy. Numerous pharmacological works have objectified the activity of these plant embryonic extracts. Birch buds have demonstrated that they can stimulate the reticuloendothelial system, the protective barrier of our body, against external aggressions. The activity of the blackcurrant bud has also been tested. This gemmotherapy increases the hormonal secretion of the adrenal cortex. It increases the resistance of laboratory animals to cold and fatigue. It makes inflammation tests negative. It is a real "cortisonelike", meaning it possesses many of the adrenal hormone properties without having the dangers, which is why it is used in rheumatism treatments. Many other buds have been studied.

That of lingonberry (Vaccinium vitis idaea), regularizes bowel movement and promotes calcium absorption, so it is used in osteoporosis. The Tilia is a non-toxic plant tranquilizer.

The young shoots of rosemary studied at the Institute of Ecology of Metz caused an increase in biliary secretion much higher than that of the adult plant. They are also capable of destroying the evil "free radicals", peroxidizing molecules which destroy cell membranes produced by an aging body. This detoxifying and anti-aging action of rosemary will be used in our various osteoarthritis treatments.

Hawthorn

Preparing the macerations

The macerations, the basis of the treatment, are preparing by macerating the fresh buds after they are picked in glycerin with alcohol. The proportion of plants is 1:20, calculated with the dehydrated weight. After 21 days, it is filtered and diluted to 1:108. Thus a glycerin maceration is obtained to the first hahnemanian decimal. That is its only dilution prescribed by the doctor. The quantity of the medication plays an important role. More concentrated, it would be too active, less and the effectiveness would be inconsistent.

Gemmotherapy against rheumatisms

In terms of rheumatology, gemmotherapy is of great importance. Due to the high activity of these buds, we can establish effective treatments without being toxic..

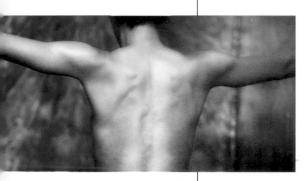

All the buds exist in drugstores in the form of drops to the first decimal. They should not be mixed with each other in the same bottle for fear of interactions decreasing their effectiveness. For osteoarthritis, no matter where located, we normally prescribe a dose of 50 to 100 drops per day of buds specific for the affliction:

Ribes nigrum buds, macerated to the first dilution (Bg Mac. 1D).

The blackcurrant bud, as we have studied it, has an anti-inflammatory action comparable to that of cortisone. But it does not have its toxic properties. Thus it does not have side effects and can be taken for long-term treatments.

Pinus Montana (Bg Mac. 1D).

The bud of the mountain pine has an analgesic and cicatrizing action on joint cartilage.

Vitis vinifera (Bg Mac. 1D).

The grape bud combats bone deformations and bone spurs of the spine. It is used in very painful deforming rheumatism as well as osteoarthritis of the fingers and toes.

To calm a lumbago

M. Charles Z., a 50 year old executive, had suffered from chronic back pain for a long time. The pain was persistent, located at the 5th lumbar vertebra and sacro-iliac joints. The ankylosis was clear: when bending the trunk without bending the knees his stretched arms out stopped at mid-thigh, stiffness was worse in the morning. Putting on his socks was a problem. The ground had never been so low for poor Mr. Z. The x-ray was unremarkable: slipping of the disk L5 S1 with pinching on the right. Large bone spurs. Blood tests confirmed that we were well within the framework of osteoarthritis. This back pain had resisted prescribed medical treatments, physical therapy even if well performed and an incredible number of manipulations. In three months of treatment (read box), we obtained practically the complete elimination of all the lumbar pain. Fairly significant physical exertions were made without triggering new attacks. His spine is more flexible, bending leads to fingers at mid-thigh and getting up has become easy.

A good example of treatment

As we wrote with our friend Dr Claude Bergeret, a good treatment program for an adult with osteoarthritis would be to drink a large glass of water a few minutes before meals for two months containing: in the morning 100 drops of *Ribes* buds Bg Mac. 1 D; at lunch 100 drops of *Pinus* Bg Mac. 1 D; at night 100 drops of *Vitis* Bg Mac. 1 D.

Other buds in rheumatology

The buds of the ash *(Fraxinus excelsior)*, apple tree *(Malus communis)*, and cherry tree *(Prunus cerasus)* are used for gout. Those of the fir *(Abies)* are remineralizing and promote growth in children. Lastly, in general terms the oak *(Quercus)* and birch *(Betula)* have an interesting anti-aging effect which is good for your joints.

Gemmotherapy in older people

Osteoarthritis in older subjects or osteoarthritis in women after menopause are more difficult to treat.

Actually, at this time of life it is necessary to take into account a significant osteoporosis, painful demineralization of the skeleton with a worrying risk of fracture, either spontaneous or after a fall. The degree of this osteoporosis and its evolution can be monitored thanks to bone mineral density measurements commonly practiced at present.

Treating osteoporosis

Also here three buds and young shoots are used:

Lingonberry, *Vaccinium vitis idaea,* which, as we have shown, improves calcium assimilation in the intestine and is anti-aging, 100 drops in the morning;

The bramble, *Rubus fructicosus,* which ensures fixation of calcium in the bone, 100 drops at lunch;

The sequoia, *Sequoia gigantea,* which increases osteo-blast activity, the bone regenerating cells. It is also anti-aging, 100 drops at dinner.

Thanks to two to three month treatments, with 50 to 100 drops daily of each one, to be repeated regularly, this formidable osteoporosis can be treated naturally. The bone remineralizes, as is possible to monitor with bone mineral density tests. Pain decreases.

Clearly, it is a good idea to pay attention to dietary intake of calcium and vitamin D at the same time, which must be sufficient.

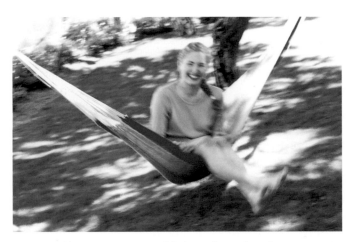

Ms. Marie D., 63 years old, has dorsolumbar osteoar-thritis with significant osteoporosis. The x-rays speak clearly. So do the bone mineral density tests. Moreover, she has a slight osteoporotic collapse of the 10th dorsal vertebra. However, Ms. D took hormone replacement treatment at menopause, which she continued for eight years and then stopped for fear of cancer when her sister was diagnosed with cancer in her left breast. Normal blood test, with, however, slightly low calcium at 87 mg/liter. Ms. D cannot take any of the traditional treat-ments which have been proposed. They cause gastritis. We prescribed the formula below for her for three months.

We alternated with three month treatments of the anti-osteoarthritis trio: Ribes, Pinus, Vitis, along with Schuss-ler cell salts for mineral intake. Over three years of treat-ment the pain disappeared and the skeleton remineralized.

HOMEOPATHY: DYNAMIC PLANTS

Homeopathy recommends numerous plants in the treatment of your rheumatisms. The results are completely remarkable.

Homeopaths will prescribe these plants not in nature as a phytotherapist would, but after a special preparation to create dilutions and above all for potentization of the dilutions to activate them. Homeopathy is a therapeutic method invented by a German doctor during the past century, Samuel Hahnemann (1755-1843). It represents a medical approach different from traditional medicine.

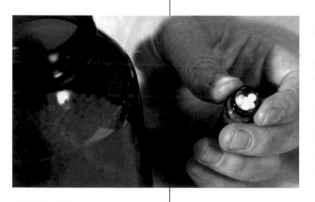

It is based on the application of a great pharmacological principle: the law of Similars- This law can be stated as follows: all substances which, administered to a healthy person, cause pathological effects, which after dilution and potentization become capable of curing similar symptoms when found in a sick person. So, for example,

At the threshold of matter

It is easy to understand, that at the heights of deconcentration of homeopathy that we are beyond ponderable and beyond the threshold of matter. And therefore, homeopathy acts outside of "placebo effect" as widely demonstrated by the great success of this method in pediatrics and veterinary medicine, as well as the interesting studies by our friend, Prof. Madeleine Bastide for example on thymulin and those of Dr. Jacques Benveniste of Inserm on the "memory of water". Homeopathy is based on an energy and therapeutic information where ponderable is only important as a starting basis for the dilutions.

Ipecac, as you well know, at high, ponderable doses is an emetic, largely used in the past. After dilution and potentization, at an infinitesimal, homeopathic dose, it becomes one of the remedies prescribed by a homeopath to treat nausea and vomiting. It is particularly useful for use in treating the frequent nausea in pregnant women at the beginning of their pregnancy, and we can prescribe the remedy without fear since there is no risk of poisoning with it nor risk of birth defects for the future baby. By the same token coffee keeps most of us from sleeping when we drink it too late in the day. This same coffee, diluted and potentized, under its Latin name *Coffea* becomes one of our remedies for insomnia.

From the plant to granules

For a plant to be used in homeopathy, experiments first need to be conducted to know its possibilities. We carry out its pathogenesis. It also needs to be diluted and potentized, with the exception of homeopathic plant mother tinctures used for drainage. Dilutions and potentizations require a series of successive codified and difficult pharmaceutical operations to be conducted by specialist pharmacists (read box). This explains why homeopathic remedies can only and will only be sold in drugstores. Most druggists are well aware of homeopathy. Take their advice.

Dilutions

There are two main techniques for preparing dilutions. The first creates dilutions above 1:100 in potentization, i.e. energetically shaking one hundred times after centesimal dilutions. This method is called Hahnemanian. Currently 4 CH, 5 CH, 7 CH, 9 CH, 12 CH, up to 30 CH. The second is called Korsakovian. It only uses one bottle subsequently filled, shaken and emptied. Its interest is to increase the vibratory energy of the potentization. This is why it is often preferred by the doctor. Currently 30xK, 200xK, 1000xK, 10000xK and 50000xK are prescribed with excellent results.

Practical homeopathy

Numerous vegetables will serve you very well in homeopathy for treating joint pain and ankyloses.

We will identify them and differentiate them based on their "procedures", i.e. the circumstances in which your pain appears or gets worse, improves or disappears – rest, movement or humidity for example. The location is also interesting. Thus we have remedies for the shoulder, elbow and knee.

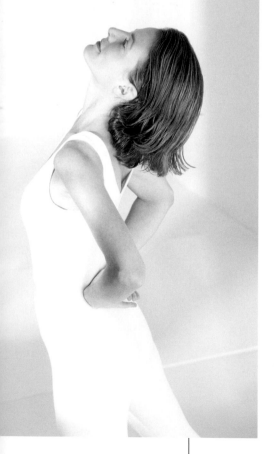

Pain when you get up

You are in pain, ankylosed and stiff in the morning when you wake up, you get better as you mobilize, you move, actually "loosening up" your joints. Here are four remedies for you:

• *Rhus toxicodendron.* This is our most important homeopathic remedy. Poison ivy, that pretty climbing plant but whose leaves can trigger eczema, is the medication for painful joint stiffness. The person suffers at the beginning of movement. gets better during the day then the pain reappears in the evening due to fatigue. The tendons and ligaments are particularly affected. The pain of patients of the Rhus tox type is also sharply aggravated by humidity. On the other hand, a dry, warm climate and locally applied heat improves it greatly. If this is your case, take 3 homeopathic granules morning and evening of Rhus tox in 30xK, far from meals, letting the grains melt slowly under your tongue.

• *Rhododendron.* From the rhododendron of the Pyrenees and Alps, this remedy is also for patients who improve with prolonged movement and worsen with humid, cold weather. But in these patients the pain is remarkably sensitive to storms. It gets significantly worse before the storm breaks and improves once it has passed. This is the Rhus tox for stormy, heavy and humid weather.

• *Ruta graveolens.* Common rue is a plant found in meadows, used in the past for its abortive properties. Homeopathically potentized, it is an excellent remedy for tendonitis and periarthritis. The flexor tendons are affected most often. You can't bend your elbow or knee. Prolonged, moderate movement improves it, as does heat. On the other hand humid cold and overworking muscles makes it worse.

• *Dulcamara.* Bittersweet, a climbing plant toxic at ponderable doses, treats problems visibly triggered by humidity. This can be neck pain, torticollis or sciatica. A change in position improves pain. Often, diarrhea alternates with the rheumatic pain.

Tell me where it hurts

The location of your rheumatism needs to be taken into consideration. Neck and upper back pain recover with *Actaea racemosa*, lumbago with *Rhus tox*, *Arnicato*. A painful shoulder is treated with Iris versicolor, the harlequin blueflag, *Sanguinaria*, the bloodroot of Canada and above all *Solanum malacoxylon* which is marvelous remedy for periarthritis of the shoulder above all in local subcutaneous injections. Hip *osteoarthritis needs Iris versicolor and Allium cepa*; knee osteoarthritis, *Bryonia*, *Phytolacca*; the small joints, above all the fingers, *Caulophyllum*, *Polygonum aviculare*, *and Actaea spicata*. All of these remedies are to use at 30xK with 3 granules 1 or 2 times per day.

Painful chronic rheumatisms

Rhus tox and *Bryonia* are the two greatest remedies for chronic rheumatisms. They complement each other well since osteoarthritis sufferers always have painful procedures in turn of the Rhus tox type and Bryonia type. In all cases of painful chronic rheumatism, the alternation of 3 granules over the long-term, will give you spectacular, long-lasting improvements: 1 day *Rhus tox* 30x K the next day *Bryonia* 30x K.

Pain with any movement

The slightest change in position causes you to cry out or at least grind your teeth. Then you require treatment with another great rheumatism remedy: *Bryonia.*

You will improve with:
- *Bryonia.* Bryony is a climbing plant frequent in hedges and undergrowth. The root, called devil's turnip, is extremely purgative.This is what homeopaths use as strain. Its homeopathic potentizations treat all rheumatisms which are worsened by the slightest movement and improve by staying completely still. Strong pressure, for example tightly holding the effected joint and local cold improves these patients. Thus *Bryonia* is used to treat neck, back and lumbar pain. Osteoarthritis of the knee with joint effusion, reacts well to Bryonia. If this is your case, take 3 granules of *Bryonia* morning and night at 30xK.

- *Phytolacca.* American pokeweed corresponds to a pain worsened by movement. The pain is searing, easily changing place, triggered by humid weather, worsening at night. This is a good remedy for sciatica, the pain which descends along the outside of the leg as if it were following the seam of your pants.

- *Ranunculus bulbosus.* The bulbous buttercup acts essentially on pain in the ribs, very sensitive to the slightest movement, light touching and humidity. It is also a good remedy for writer's cramp, which affects the forearm and hand of rheumatics.

Joints deformed by gout

These joints, with the presence of uric acid tophus can also be treated by homeopathy.

You can try:

• *Colchicum.* Autumn crocus blooms in fall. Its bulb is picked at the beginning of summer.

Its gout-fighting action is due to the presence of cholchicine, an alkaloid with very well known anti-uric properties. The remedy in ponderable doses may be preferred during an acute attack, along with anti-inflammatory drugs. But this does not prevent a repetition of the attacks unlike long-terms daily doses of 3 granules of *Colchicum* 30xK. Painful feet are relieved by applications of heat. This procedure allows rapid differentiation with a second great homeopathic remedy for gout, *Ledum palustre.*

• *Ledum.* The "marsh Labrador tea" type patient actually has the peculiarity of being relieved by the cold. The eminent American homeopath James Tyler Kent often told his colleagues a story which illustrates well this peculiarity of ledon. Called for an emergency to a notary public's who had a violent attack of gout, he found the wounded notary with his feet plunged halfway up his calf in a bucket of water with numerous ice cubes floating in it. "See this is the only way I can find to get rid of my pain", exclaimed the patient when Kent arrived. "*Ledum* 10 000x K", the homeopath replied to him. One single dose and the notary no longer suffered. *Ledum* does not always give such spectacular results. But 3 granules morning and night, more modestly at 30x K, will help you get your toes moving again.

Lignum vitae

Guaiacum is also a good remedy for gout-related arthritis. Just as for *Ledum*, the patient feels better thanks to contact with cold, and oddly enough, when eating apples. There are numerous tophus with significant joint deformities.

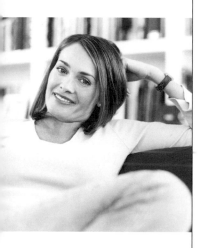

Glucosamine

A few years back an American researcher published a study reporting the astonishing effectiveness of a substance in repairing cartilage damaged in osteoarthritis: glucosamine. This treatment has been used for a few years.

Glucosamine is part of the molecules that build the cartilage structure which plays an essential role, by absorbing and ejecting the synovial fluid contained in joints. Glucosamine acts on different levels:

• it stimulates cartilage synthesis;
• it acts against inflammation;
• it stimulates repair phenomena.
All of these actions contribute to effectively fight the symptoms of osteoarthritis and inflamed joints: pain, stiffness and inflammation.

Scientific proof

Numerous studies have evaluated the effectiveness of glucosamine for treating osteoarthritis starting in the 1960's. The longest, and thus most convincing was published in 2001 in the famous English medical journal Lancet. Researchers from the University of Liège divided 212 osteoarthritis patients into two groups: the first received a daily dose of 1,500 mg of glucosamine sulfate for three years and the second a placebo. The researchers then took x-rays of the knees of patients under stress one year and three years after the treatment started. They found a significant reduction in the space between the knee bones in the patients taking the placebo. This reduction of 0.31 mm demonstrated the progression of the disease. But, this space remained stable in the patients treated with glucosamine. In this group, the symptoms improved 25% on average and they worsened in the placebo group. In several studies, glucosamine improved the symptoms of osteoarthritis of the knee, vertebrae, hips and shoulders. This improvement was found from the end of a six week treatment and confirmed 2 weeks after it was stopped. Over the long term, the improvement continued in the treated osteoarthritis patients. Moreover, and far from being unimportant, the x-rays show that the cartilage destruction process was stabilized. The disease no longer progressed. Glucosamine is well tolerated: a few stomach problems such as heartburn, stomachache or diarrhea may appear but they disappear when the treatment is stopped.

Better than anti-inflammatory drugs

The effectiveness and tolerance of glucosamine has been compared to that of nonsteroidal anti-inflammatory drugs. Glucosamine appears to be as effective as ibuprofen given at the dose of 1.5 grams per day for the first and 1.2 grams per day for the second. In another study, glucosamine continued to act for several weeks after treatment was stopped, unlike ibuprofen. Moreover, glucosame was better tolerated that the anti-inflammatory drug with fewer side effects.

A few precautions for using it

LGlucosamine sulfate does have some contraindications all the same. Diabetics should not take it. The treatment requires monitoring by a physician if you are allergic to shellfish. Glucosamine is often "wrapped" in crab shell which can cause allergies.

Antioxidants

Numerous antioxidant substances, especially vitamins, have proven their effectiveness in treating osteoarthritis: they are used to slow down the progression of the disease.

As soon as the cartilage starts to become damaged and crack the destruction process is increased by the resulting inflammation. The disease take hold. The only way of really acting on the disease is to supply the body with substances able to stop the activity of the destructive enzymes. This is the role of antioxidants, substances produced by the body (glutathione) or obtained through the diet (vitamins C and E, selenium and carotenoids) to protect the cells from aging. Some of these have a particularly effective action on joints.

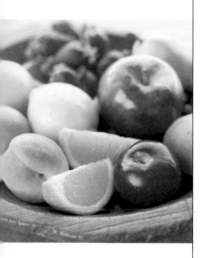

Vitamin C

The *Framingham Osteoarthritis Cohort Study,* an American study conducted on 640 people, showed that vitamin C protects against osteoarthritis. The participants filled in questionnaires on their diets and their consumption of supplements. Researchers followed the evolution of their

The role of selenium

Selenium is a mineral found in the soil and which we get from the fruits and vegetables we eat. A powerful antioxidant, it is stored in the muscles and liver and plays an essential role in the body. Unfortunately, blood levels decrease with age, and we, American, are pretty badly off since our soil is especially poor in selenium. It is also indispensable for the production of certain cartilage substances. A selenium deficiency causes an alteration of these cells and by repercussion a lack of collagen in the cartilage. A favorable context for progression of the disease.

joints and knees for around 10 years. Of the people who ate the most vitamin C, between 152 and 430 mg per day, i.e. 4 times the recommended amount for an adult, the osteoarthritis progressed 3 times slower than in the people who consumed the least. To obtain 430 mg per day, you need to take a supplement. In July 2003, Niels Jensen, a general practitioner from Copenhagen showed that daily tablets of 2g of vitamin C reduced pain and improved movement in people affected with osteoarthritis of the knee or hip. 133 people took vitamin C then the placebo (or vice versa but without knowing) for 2 periods of 15 days.

Vitamin E

Since 1978 several scientific studies have shown that vitamin E supplements make it possible to reduce pain and decrease the amount of medication taken. However other more recent studies have not found great benefits.

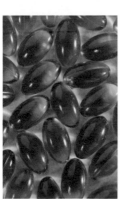

Vitamin E is probably more effective when associated with other antioxidants like vitamin C, carotenoids and selenium. This is what a recent study on animals suggests: a food supplement with these antioxidants made it possible to prevent osteoarthritis in mice which are genetically weak from an osteoarticular viewpoint.

Free radicals, antioxidants... what are they?

Oxygen is the main fuel of the human body ...and paradoxically also the main cause of its aging. The use of oxygen by the cells generates waste, the famous free radicals, toxic for the body. Pollution and tobacco are also sources of free radicals which modify the genetic code of cells, and change their correct functioning. To protect itself, the body also produces enzymes capable of neutralizing them. It can also use antioxidant substances that it finds in food. If these antioxidant reserves are not sufficient, the free radicals accumulate and contribute to cell destruction.

Focus on selenium

It was long believed dangerous. But this trace element is one of our most effective weapons against free radicals.

What is it?

Selenium is a trace element present in the soil. It is taken up by plants which transform it into a compound which can be assimilated by our body, such as selenomethoinine. It enters the food chain. Even though this mineral is present in very low quantities in our body it is indispensable for living. The concentration of selenium in the soil varies greatly based on the region. For example, in Ohio where the soil is very poor in selenium the cancer rate is two times higher than Dakota where the ground is particularly rich.

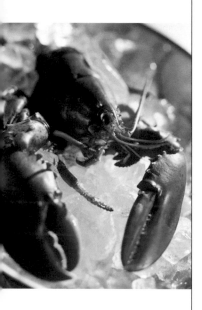

What is it used for?

First of all it is an antioxidant, i.e. it fights the harmful action of free radicals. Actually, it is needed for glutathione peroxidase (GPx) to work. This enzyme which is present in our body is part of our internal defense system against free radicals. If you lack selenium, your GPx enzymes do not work well and you cannot effectively protect yourself against free radicals. In the long term a low rate of GPx may increase the risk for cardiovascular diseases. An American study on 30,000 people which lasted twelve years showed that a daily selenium supplement makes it possible to decrease the risks of lung, esophagus, colon, and above all, prostate cancer. Selenium is also more effective when it is associated with other antioxidants such as vitamin E. An NPC (Nutritional Prevention of Cancer) study demonstrated that selenium supplementation reduces cancer mortality by

50%. Selenium also protects the immune system, improves the production and motility of sperm, helps to thin blood and contributes to eliminating toxic products such as mercury or lead, and lastly, possesses anti-inflammatory properties. But it can become toxic if present in too high quantities in the body.

How much is necessary?

Daily needs are around 60 mcg (micrograms) for women and 80 mcg for men, but numerous studies have suggested that it is necessary to take 100 to 200 mcg per day for the best antioxidant effectiveness. Amounts less than 30 mcg/day lead to a deficiency and serious consequences for the heart. The average amount taken in through the diet is around 45 mcg/day, leading to the need to take supplements.

Is there a risk of overdose?

In high doses, selenium is a poison. Inhalation of powders or fumes rich in selenium in certain industries can cause acute intoxication: headache, nausea, vomiting and eye and skin problems. Moreover, certain selenium-rich shampoos should be used prudently especially with children. On the other hand, food is rarely the cause of an overdose. According to studies, doses of around 500 mcg/day do not cause any problems.

Main sources of selenium (mcg/100g)

Barley	70
Oysters, lobster	65
Bread	27
Eggs	20
Mushrooms	13
Chicken	10
Cheese	9
Carrots	2

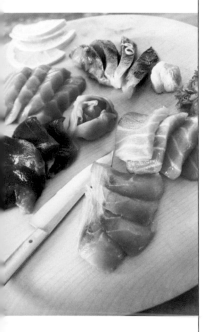

Omega-3: fish oils to fight inflammation

Fatty fish oils are rich in omega-3 fats which have an anti-inflammatory action proven many times over.

On the tracks of the Eskimos

The first report on the medical interest in cod liver oil was published in the *London Medical Journal* in… 1783! More recently, in 1980, Danish researchers realized that inflammatory diseases (particularly joint and cardiovascular) are much rarer in Eskimos than the rest of the world. It was their diet which put the scientists on the right track: the Eskimos are the biggest consumers of fatty fish. These animals contribute fats of a special type called omega-3. Omega-3 when eaten, give rise to substances in the body which discourage inflammation. This resulted in the idea of giving fish oils to treat inflammatory diseases. Since then numerous clinical studies have proven the effectiveness of fish oils for treating inflammatory joint diseases, especially rheumatoid arthritis, but also osteoarthritis or psoriatic arthritis. The results show that patients who take gel capsules of fish oil on a daily basis (generally 3 g/day for rheumatoid arthritis) have less pain in the affected joints and can move better after 3 months of treatment than those who take a placebo.

Protecting the cartilage

Omega-3 makes it possible to slow down, or even stop, the activity of the cells involved in the cartilage inflam-

Where can I buy fish oils?

Fish oils are sold in the form of food supplements or medications at drug stores (capsules, gel capsules). They are assimilated perfectly by the body. They should be taken at night since cells regenerate during the night. Ask your pharmacist for advice.

mation and destruction process. By limiting cartilage destruction, the evolution of the disease can be mitigated and the joints preserved for a longer time. In 1989, the first study on osteoarthritis demonstrated that 10 ml cod liver oil per day led to an improvement of mobility and pain after 6 weeks of treatment. It is interesting to note that in this study, olive oil (also anti-inflammatory) obtained similar results. If the studies on omega-3 were mainly conducted on people afflicted with rheumatoid arthritis, more recently obtained results and knowledge on the way omega-3 fatty acids act on cartilage show that people who have osteoarthritis can also benefit from this treatment.

Where does omega-3 come from?

Omega-3 fats are obtained from food: they are primarily found in nuts, linseed, green vegetables and canola and nut oils. But, also in animals products from animals fed flax (eggs, certain meats) and in fatty fish (salmon, herring, sardine and mackerel). The current diet contains less and less due to the massive consumption of a family of antagonist and proinflammatory fats, omega-6, which are found in sunflower and corn oils, and in the meat of corn-fed animals. Modern diets, poor in omega-3 and overly rich in omega-6, contribute to inflammatory diseases.

To prevent cardiovascular diseases as well!

Omega-3 has been widely studies, and used, to prevent heart attacks. It actually lowers the level of triglycerides in the blood (a cardiovascular risk factor) and thins the blood at the same time. Since the beginning of the 1990's numerous studies have shown that cardiac patients who eat more fat rich in omega-3, in the form of canola oil or margarine, in fish, or in fish oil capsules, decrease their risk of heart attack.

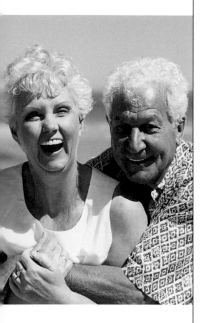

Vitamin D

We have all benefited from vitamin D supplements as children, especially during the long winter months, to prevent rickets. This disease has been known since the 17th century and in 1782 doctors noticed the protective role of cod liver oil which is rich in vitamin D.

What is vitamin D used for?

It helps the bones to stay solid and rigid (prevention of rickets in children and osteoporosis in adults). Vitamin D acts on the bones by regulating the metabolism of calcium and promoting its fixation. The administration of vitamin D is systematic for newborns and infants above all those who are not exposed to the sun (winter months, ethnical customs). It regulates immunity: many studies suggest that it may prevent autoimmune diseases such as insulin-dependant diabetes in children. It also possesses an anti-cancer power.

Finding and preserving vitamin D

Our body has two ways of obtaining this vitamin:
• By exposure to the sun: the skin synthesizes vitamin D from cholesterol, under the influence of ultraviolet rays. This is the main source but it depends on the amount of sunshine and the season. It is practically impossible to produce vitamin D between November and February, even if you are exposed to the sun.
• From the diet: cod liver oil is hardly taken any more. Dietary vitamin D comes from fatty fish, yolk, liver and dairy products. Vitamin D2 in the form of drops (but not in the form of ampoules) are sold over the counter in drugstores as well as vitamin D ointments. Vitamin D3, the most active and thus most interesting, is by prescription.

What are the signs of a deficiency?

Vitamin D deficiencies are the most frequent in the elderly. In children a deficiency leads to rickets with bone swelling and deformities and in adults to osteomalacia with bone and muscle pain. Deficiencies effect 75% of adults living in cities during the winter. This can contribute to osteoporosis and its fractures and increase the risk of colon, breast, prostate and skin (melanoma) cancer.

Is too much vitamin D dangerous?

High (more than 40,000 IU/day) and prolonged doses of vitamin D can cause hypercalcemia with nausea, headaches and loss of appetite. Over time, calcium may be deposited in the tissue. A dose of 2,000 to 4,000 IU/day is a reasonable threshold which should not be exceeded. Vitamin D synthesized by the sun is not toxic, but too much sun is not good for you either!

Average vitamin D contents in certain foods
(µg per 100 g)

Cod liver oil	250 to 750
Sardines	36
Tuna	25
Salmon	5
Egg (yolk)	2 to 12
Cow milk	2
Butter	2
Comté, gruyere	1
Breast milk	1

Special vitamin D meals for long winter nights

Steamed salmon
or sardines,
a portion of Comté
and floating islands

Who needs vitamin D supplements?

Doses from 400 to 800 IU/day can be proposed to the following categories:

• Infants.

• Children and adolescents in particular from October to March.

• City dwellers, from October to March.
• Seniors especially over age 65.
• People who live in polluted cities (decrease in ultraviolet rays) or in regions with not much sunlight.
• Pregnant women or nursing mothers (under a physician's care).
• People with a risk of cancer of the colon (family history or existing polyps), breast (family cases, mastitis) and prostate (high PSA level).

High doses under a physician's care can be proposed to the following individuals:

• Cancer patients, as an adjuvant treatment (mainly synthetic analogues of vitamin D are administered).
• People with rickets, osteoporosis or osteomalacia.
• Subjects treated with certain medications such as cortisone, laxatives and barbiturates.

Who should avoid taking it?

Patients with hyperthyμorders and diseases interfering with calcium metabolism. All people treated for a disease which causes hypercalcemia.
People who are sensitive to vitamin D.

What are our daily needs?

They are measured in international units (IU) and more recently in micrograms (μg):

$$1 \text{ IU} = 0.025 \text{ μg or } 1 \text{ μg} = 40 \text{ IU}$$

Vitamin D can be measured in the blood, it is mainly stored in fatty tissue. Numerous specialists feel that the recommended amounts in the US are insufficient. The leading specialist in the world, Professor Reinhold Vieth (University of Toronto) estimates that this should be multiplied by at least 2 and maybe by 5 in adults. The needs are rarely satisfied. For this reason, before starting treatments under a physician's care, it is important to get dietary advice for a correct management of vitamin D, particularly by regularly eating fatty fish and regular exposure to sunlight.

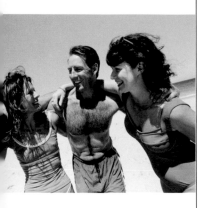

Vitamin K

We are more familiar with its antagonists (anti-vitamin K or anticoagulants) prescribed when there is a risk of thrombosis or embolism, or after a heart attack.

What is vitamin K used for?

Known since 1929 for its anti-hemorrhage action, it was isolated in 1936 and synthesized in 1939. It was later learned that vitamin K helps fix calcium on bones. This is why it is of interest in association with vitamin D in osteoporosis.

Finding and preserving vitamin K

Vitamin K is found in most of our foods. Green leafy vegetables (cabbage, parsley, spinach and broccoli) contain the most, especially when fresh. Vitamin K is destroyed by light but stable with heat and not soluble in water: losses from cooking are minimal.

When there is a vitamin K deficiency

There are 3 vitamin K:
• K1 obtained from vegetables;
• K2 synthesized in the body by intestinal bacteria;
• K3 which is the synthetic form.
Deficiencies are rare. On the other hand, premature babies and newborns are threatened since breast milk is low in vitamin K and their intestinal bacteria cannot produce it.

A vitamin K deficiency can cause hemorrhages leading to anemia.

Vitamin K likes

(INCREASED EFFECTIVENESS)
Calcium and vitamin D

Vitamin K does not like

(DECREASED EFFECTIVENESS)
Anticoagulants, iron, an excess of vitamins A and E, aspirin and medications like some antibiotics and seizure medications

Is too much vitamin K dangerous?

Vitamins K1 and K2 are not very dangerous. Excessive doses of vitamin K3 can destroy red blood cells causing anemia. In some countries, vitamin K supplements are not authorized as food supplements and are considered similar to medications.

Who needs vitamin K supplements

• Premature babies and newborns.
• Infants who are only breastfed.

Your vitamin K needs will increase if:
• You have chronic digestion problems.
• You have to undergo an operation with the risk of hemorrhage.
• You are pregnant or nursing.
• You are in menopause or elderly.

Who should not take it?

Patients being treated with anticoagulants.

What are our daily needs?

They are measured in micrograms (μg) of vitamin K. Blood tests are not usual, deficiencies are detected by checking the blood coagulation function.

A K filled meal

Lettuce, sauerkraut with meat, strawberry or peach

Vitamin E

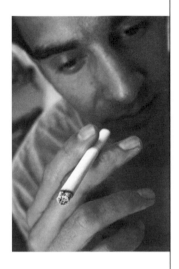

What is vitamin E used for?

Discovered in 1920, synthesized in 1928, its very interesting properties have been known since 1970. Before that, this vitamins was used for childless couples, especially to increase the sperm count in men – a use not based on any scientific reality. The same is not true for the areas for which it is now known: prevention of cardiovascular diseases and cancer. Since vitamin E is an antioxidant: it works hand in hand with beta carotene and vitamin C against free radicals. Its role: to protect against oxidation of the body's fat.

Finding and preserving vitamin E

It is from oleaginous plants (almonds and walnuts) and virgin or extra-virgin vegetable oils that we get most of our vitamin E, especially from sunflower oil. Generally, all foods rich in polyunsaturated fat are rich in vitamin E But they use it themselves first in order not to go rancid, supplying our body with minimal amounts, which is the reason for supplements. Vitamin E is sensitive to the light (keep oil in an opaque bottle). When cooked it loses an estimated 20%.

What are the signs of a deficiency?

There is no disease caused by a vitamin E deficiency: one can have a major deficiency without any symptoms. Four people out of ten receive two thirds of the minimum recommended daily amounts.

Is too much vitamin E dangerous?

Vitamin E is atoxic. Medications with vitamin E generally containing 500 mg (500 IU) can be taken daily without problems. However, care needs to be taken with people who have a tendency to bleed or who are on anticoagulants, since vitamin E thins the blood.

Who needs vitamin E supplements?

Vitamin can be considered beneficial for all humans, it improves immunity, protects against the number of malignant tumors and cardiovascular complications.

Average vitamin E contents in certain foods (mg/100g)

Wheat germ oil	160
Walnut oil	63
Sunflower oil	60
Peanut oil	25
Olive oil	10
Cod liver oil	22
Margarine	15 to 40
Wheat germ	149
Almonds, hazel nuts	45
Peanuts	10

You should consider taking a daily vitamin E supplement (50 to 200 mg):
• If you smoke. Vitamin E has a depolluting role and protects against arteriosclerosis.
• If you have a high risk of prostate cancer, one study demonstrated a 30% decreased risk in smokers who took supplements.
• If you drink too much, alcohol increases free radicals.
• If you are diabetic, to decrease the risk of complications.
• If you have heart disease and you have a risk of thrombosis.
• If you want to slow down aging and prevent certain complications, starting from middle age.
• If you are a carrier of an allergy or an autoimmune disease.
• If you have had a kidney transplant.
• If you have had chemotherapy or radiation treatments.

- If you practice a sport intensively.
- If you are chronically exposed to pollution.
- If you have to be exposed to sunlight.
- If you live at a high altitude.
- If you have cirrhosis of the liver.
- If you are being treated with anti-psychotics.
- If you take oral contraceptives

Who should avoid taking high does?

- During the last month of pregnancy.
- Before surgery.
- In cases of bleeding due to coagulation problems.
- After a cerebral hemorrhage.
- In cases of retinitis pigmentosa, and genetic diseases affecting the retina.

What are our daily needs?

They are measured in international units (IU) and in alpha-tocopherol equivalents (alpha-TE).

1 mg of synthetic vitamin E (dl-alpha-tocopherol) = 1 IU
1 mg of natural vitamin E (d-alpha-tocopherol) =
1 alpha-TE = 1.49 IU
Alpha-tocopherol can be measured in the blood, although most of our vitamin E is found in fatty tissue.

Vitamin E likes (INCREASED EFFECTIVENESS)	Vitamin E does not like (DECREASED EFFECTIVENESS)
vitamin C	paraffin oil
selenium	iron
carotenoids	copper
	the contraceptive pill

Selecting a vitamin E supplement

The term vitamin E applies to several substances: four tocopherols (alpha, beta, gamma, delta) and four tocotrienols (alpha, beta, gamma, delta). Most of the supplements sold are in the form of alpha-tocopherol. The natural form (d-alpha) seems more effective than the synthetic form (dlalpha). However, if one believes recent works, gamma-tocopherol (the most widespread in foods) is preferable to alpha-tocopherol. The ideal is definitely a mix of natural tocopherols and tocotrienols .

Vitamin E and the heart

Two types of studies associate vitamin E and cardiovascular prevention: epidemiology studies (observation) and intervention studies, where the vitamin is compared to a placebo.

In two epidemiology studies on more than 100,000 people, those who took a vitamin E supplement had a 40% lower cardiac risk. A study conducted on 11,000 elderly people demonstrated that users of vitamin C and vitamin E supplements had a 53% lower cardiovascular mortality risk. Four intervention studies have been conducted. In the CHAOS study, the supplements reduced the number of non-fatal heart attacks by 77% in people with heart disease. In the GISSI study, the group of heart patients who took vitamin E had half of the deaths of those who took a placebo. On the other had, the other two studies did not find any benefits.

Trace elements

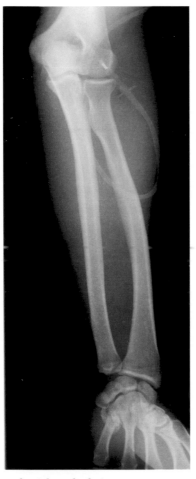

More and more people suffer from osteoarthritis pain, numerous patients take anti-inflammatory drugs practically in continuation, which does not fail to cause inconveniences (gastric pain and bleeding). There is a very high demand for natural medicine medications.

Phytotherapy is the first choice, no therapist can skip Harpagophytum, meadowsweet and blackcurrant among others. Acupuncture and auriculotherapy are equally effective and combine very well with an oral treatment. Oligotherapy has an undeniable place. Its highly manageable nature makes it possible for it to supplement all the other methods.

The most used trace elements include:
• phosphorus: one of the constituents of the mineral substance of bone;
• sulfur: an element making up the cartilage, which explains the interest in chondroitins sulfates for treating osteoarthritis of the knee;
• le silicon: indispensable for bone calcification and growth. Readily available in vegetable form, horsetail, bamboo or nettle gel capsules;
• manganese: plays a role in the synthesis of the essential constituents of cartilage, often associated with cobalt in a manganese cobalt compound;
• copper: important role in the mechanisms that fight inflammation;
• fluorine: in the event of osteoporosis associated to osteoarthritis processes.

Basic treatment for osteoarthritis:

• Manganese cobalt: once a day every day.
• Sulfur: once a day every other day.
• Silicon treatment (bamboo gel capsules 15 days per month).
• Possibly potassium and magnesium: two times per week.
• In the event of an acute worsening, copper is indispensable: two to three times per day.

For osteoporosis, fluorine can be added to the basic treatment. In the trace element form, fluorine does not cause any problems of a weight gain. Modern osteoporosis treatments are not harmless and the warnings have multiplied. The generalization and reimbursement of the bone mineral density testing makes it possible to discover a number of "borderline" osteoporosis cases but which will automatically be treated with biphosphonates, renalates or another miraculous product. Wouldn't it be better to start with less aggressive treatments? Do the possible long-term benefits compensate the problems? Moreover, do they know everything at present? These different therapeutic schemes can be adapted and modified. Each therapist has his or her habits and is interested in innovation, especially in the case of total or partial failure.

No matter what, if a basic treatment is started, it must last several months.

The latest research

Recent studies have shown that certain nutriments in our diet have a remarkable importance for keeping joints intact. They are not found in all diets and often need to be added with supplements.

Osteoarthritis is a joint aging process which starts by altering and then destroying the cartilage that covers and lubricates our joints. Bone demineralization and deformities are second only to changes in the cartilage. The cartilage disease comes before the bone disease. Some nutrients are especially interesting for stopping this process.

Medications and supplements have been created which are integrated with a modern nutritional therapy approach to osteoarthritis. These are substances which normally exist in our skeleton and which, except for bravely crunching if you have good teeth, chicken and fish bones, are not part of our menus. Thus they must be taken in other forms.

Cartilage, crabs and lobsters

Chondroitin sulfuric acid (C.S.A.), its sodium salt to be precise, one of the essential constituents of joint cartilage, has been isolated. Administered orally in 3 gel capsules per day, it exercises an anti-osteoarthritis action over the long-term. But it is necessary to take prolonged treatments to observe a positive effect.

C.S.A. decreases the activity of an enzyme, elastase, an agent which destroys joint cartilage and then stops its destruction. On the other hand, it stimulates the secretion of sulfur proteins, the proteoglycans processed by the cartilage cells or chondrocytes, cicatrizing observed destruction. These proteoglycans play an important role in hydration of joint collagen thus in maintaining supple tissue in your knees or nape.

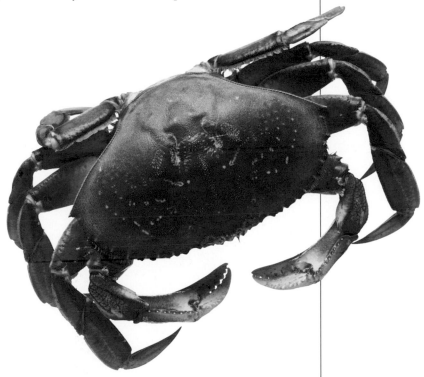

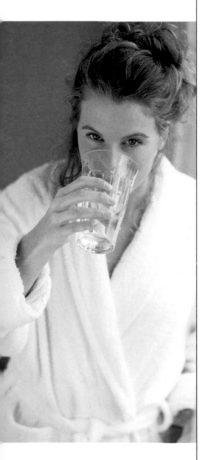

SPA TREATMENT
The patient

Spa treatments are no longer just a trend. Their health benefits have long been recognized. And the medical community uses them as a global therapeutic means. So much the better for the patient since they are so pleasant.

A spa treatment is a complex group of treatments dedicated to harmony and peacefulness. The treatment does not just involve care ...but also an environmental and human approach. Nature, the architecture and interior decoration are small important details. They extend the "zen" ambiance distilled by healthcare personnel. From the reception to leisure time, dialogue is vital for making patients feel at ease. It is important to undergo treatment for several years in a row to take advantage of the benefits. Most often, a three week treatment is repeated three years in a row. The spa is selected based on the patient's disease, special spa treatments and the geographical location, easy for the patient to get to.

How does it work step by step?

The patient will be given a schedule including the treatment times: baths, showers, massages, application of mud, rehabilitation, etc. These treatments can be tiring, so the day is organized so that the patient has time to rest. In addition to these treatments, it is advisable to drink plenty and regularly during the day to get the most from the benefits of the thermal water. Spa treatments are recognized as a medical resource for fighting diseases and illnesses. The National Public Health Service thus pays for spa treatments. On one condition: the pathology you have must be on a list of afflictions for which a spa treatment may lead to improvement. This is the case for numerous rheumatisms, and especially osteoarthritis.

Conquering neuralgia

Neuralgia is pain of a neurological origin: it is due to the compression of a nerve by bone deformities, especially bone spurs, which causes osteoarthritis. Warm baths and applications of very hot mud proposed by spas are excellent for this type of problem.

Mineral waters for all tastes!

• Sulfur based waters have an action against rheumatisms. They also fight against bacteria of the respiratory tract mucous membranes.
• Sulfate based waters act on the kidneys, digestive tract, liver and gall bladder.
• Chlorinated waters, similar to sea water, are interesting for functional rehabilitation of joints
after an operation or in the event of an accident. They are also used for nervous or gynecological disorders.
• Lastly, cardiovascular and dermatological diseases are improved thanks to bicarbonated waters, just like allergies!

Since Antiquity...

The remains of Roman baths prove the use of spas since ancient times. However, it was in 1604, during the reign of Henry IV that the first Charte des eaux thermales (spa map) was enacted in France. During the 18th century spring water was analyzed and classified based on its properties. To be used as a mineral water, spring water must now have an authorization from the Ministry of Public Health, which is assisted by recommendations from the National Academy of Medicine.

The benefits for rheumatisms

Spa mud and water are used at a high temperature to relieve joint pain and stiffness. It is the heat, along with the minerals which provide a beneficial action.

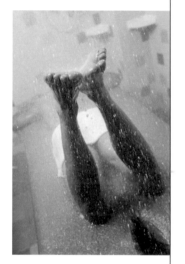

Of all the joint rheumatisms, it is osteoarthritis which gets the most benefit from a spa treatment. The aim of the treatment is to relieve pain and recover better joint mobility. The baths and the muds with hot mineral water decrease the damaging manifestations of the disease. They spread their heat to the body and improve muscle relaxation. The heat also has the property of decreasing pain and improving local circulation. The vitality of the tissues which serve to support and act as a hinge between the different elements (muscles and cartilage) around the joints is also stimulated. Reinforced thanks to the baths and mud, the peripheral tissues can then fully play their role and relieve the joints. One can decide whether to take the baths or showers, or even combine them. Spas also propose massages thanks to

3 weeks of treatment, 6 months of benefits

A French study conducted in 1997 at Vichy showed that a spa treatment of 3 weeks made it possible to decrease joint pain and anti-inflammatory drugs doses for people affected with osteoarthritis of the hip, knee or back (lumbar) for the following 6 months. Mobility and quality of life are improved, as is all mobility. In 2002 a German study showed that the baths with sulfur water also made it possible for 19 people suffering from osteoarthritis to reduce the progression of the disease.

the powerful flow of mineral water aimed at the body. The treatment program includes physical therapy sessions, to maintain joint mobility. A spa treatment is also an opportunity for following a low calorie diet, since excess weight is an aggravating factor of osteoarthritis.

And the other rheumatisms?

Doctors have long wondered about the effectiveness of spa treatments on inflammatory rheumatisms. The treatment is wise only for some people. In those who suffer from a polyarthritis of the limbs, mobilization in an environment with spa steam may sometimes lead to an astonishing recovery!! But it is necessary to admit that the results arenot as good on people suffering from joint rheumatic diseases which have an inflammatory origin (like ankylosing spondylitis and bacterial arthritis). They are less consistent for osteoarthritis. Cases of gout and psoriasis, which may be responsible for rheumatisms are treated in some spas. For all diseases, it is contraindicated to undergo a spa treatment during an inflammatory surge of the disease.

Mud...

The joints affected by osteoarthritis are coated with a thick layer of mud which is left on for ten minutes or so. The mud stays at a temperature 10 to 20° higher than body temperature. The aim is to allow the exchange of minerals (calcium and trace elements) and penetration of biological substances The type of substances depends on the type of water. Typical example: seaweed, whose benefits are widely recognized, at spas located near the ocean. This use of mud is called "illutation".

Physical therapy, an indispensable supplement

Physical therapy is an essential supplement to the treatment. The physical therapist manipulates the limbs affected by rheumatisms: he himself performs movements to make the joint work gently. Then it is the person who performs the movements actively to make their joints work.ons.

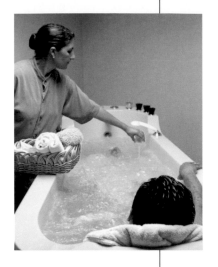

Hydrotherapy at home

Phytotherapy lets you prepare effective baths, for the entire body or parts of the body.

There are local, targeted baths developed and advocated in particular by the Abbot Sebastian Kneipp. There are also medical baths for the feet, footbaths and baths of the arms. Sitz baths were created by Dr. Kuhn, cold baths, highly ridiculed by the ignorant, however endowed with a wonderful activity on general tone, good for women as well as men since they stimulate, the master Yang point of the entire body according to acupuncturists. In terms of baths, personal sensitivity to hot water always needs to be considered. First you start with a minimum temperature, 25°C for example, and gradually progress to 30°C. You start with a shorter bath. An anti-rheumatic bath is taken normally in the morning, with the occasional exception.

To prepare these baths, you use an infusion of plants or a decoction prepared by boiling the plant, or both.

Bathtub or bowl

A complete bath in a normal bathtub uses 300 quarts of water for an adult. It reaches the level of the bathtub overflow. A half-bath represents 150 to 200 quarts, a bidet or a large basin, 30 to 50 quarts. The concentration of medicinal plants you need for your medical bath are based on these quantities.

Of pains and baths

The main formulas we recommend if you suffer from osteoarthritis, no matter where located, are as follows:

- **The mixed – anti-inflammatory heather bath** *(to mix)*:

Heather (flowery tops) 50 g ; pine (needles) 100 g ; birch (leaves) 100 g. Steep the entire mixture for 10 minutes in 2 quarts of boiling water. Filter, and add to the bath water. These trees and flowers are excellent for relieving congestion in painful joints, particularly the hips and sacro-iliac joints.

- **The mixed – de-ankylosizing horseweed bath -** *(to mix)*:

Horseweed (tops) 50 g; couch grass (roots) 50 g; black-currant (leaves) 50 g; solidago 50 g. Let steep for 10 minutes in 2 quarts of boiling water, filter, and add to the bath water. Interesting for relieving ankylosis of stiff joints, particularly the shoulders and knees.

- **The mixed – vascular tonic horse chestnut bath** *(to mix)*:

Horse chestnut (bark) 50 g; red vine (leaves) 50 g; hazel (leaves) 50 g; hamamelis 50 g. Steep for 15 minutes in 2 quarts of boiling water, filter and add to the bath water. This bath activates vein and artery circulation around locked joints. It fights osteoarthritis by stimulating blood circulation. It is excellent for hip osteoarthritis.

Bath temperature: be careful

We recommend mainly luke-warm baths from 25°C to 30°C with sometimes a hot bath at 32°C taking into consideration the person's sensation of cold. Baths which are too hot are dange-rous especially for those with heart disease. They require attentive and constant moni-toring. Someone needs to stay near the bathtub. A bath lasts 5 to 15 minutes. A bath always needs to be followed by a period of rest lying down of the same duration.

They are used for gentle massages 2 to 3 times a day
- Lavender oil:
let 40 g of fresh flowers steep for 4 days in 1 quart of olive oil and filter.
- Heather oil:
steep 50 g of flowery tops for 10 days in 1 quart of olive oil, filter.
- St. John's wort oil:
more complicated to prepare, according to Dr. Leclerc's formula:
steep 500 g of freshly picked flowery tops for 3 days in a mixture of 1 quart of olive oil and a pint of white wine vinegar. The boil in a double-boiler until the wine evaporates. You will obtain a liquor with a wonderful crimson color. Soak some gauze compresses and cover the affected part. This analgesic salve is also cicatrizing.

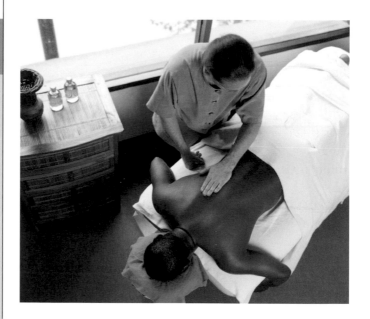

• **The mixed – analgesic willow bath** *(to mix)*: White willow (stem bark) 50 g; meadowsweet (flowery tops) 50 g; blackcurrant (leaves) 50 g. Steep for 10 minutes in 2 quarts of water, filter and add to the bath water. Very analgesic, also sudorific, it is useful for all spinal osteoarthritis pain, especially cervical.

• **Seaweed bath – joint rejuvenation***(to mix)*: Fucus 100 g; laminaires 100 g.
Fucus 100 g; laminars 100 g. Boil for 10 minutes in 2 quarts of water, filter over a large gage sieve, this decoction will be viscous due to the seaweed. Add to lukewarm bath water. De-ankylosizing, it eliminates the cellulite of affected joints. Good for the knees and lumbar area, but it stains the bathtub. To be taken in the morning, since it is irritating at night.

For the hands and feet

Two local baths acts on deformities and pain in the fingers, toes, metatarsal, tarsal, heel bone and astragalus:

- **Mixed oak footbath** – for your painful, swollen feet with toes that are killing you *(to mix)*: Oak (bark) 20 g; willow (bark) 20 g; thyme (flowery tops) 10 g; rosemary (branches) 10 g. Let it bubble 15 or 20 minutes while you relax.

- **Aromatic labiate hand bath** – for your deformed Oregano (flowery tops) 5 g; rosemary (branches) 5 g; thyme (flowery tops) 5 g; wild thyme (flowery tops) 5 g. Boil for 10 minutes in a pint of water, filter and and add to the water in your basin. Soak your hands, wrists and forearms for 10 minutes at 35°C. All of these baths are to be taken three times a week. The complete bath should be taken either one hour before meals, or two hours after. People with heart disease, high blood pressure or who are too tired should refrain.

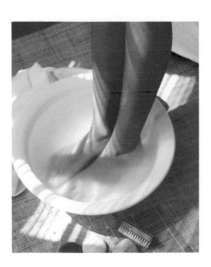

Local treatment complete the action of these baths. They are aimed at acting directly on the affected joint with a slightly revulsive action. Poultices, aromatic oils and liniments will also stimulate *(read box)*.

Poultices

These are applied on the painful joint, above all shoulders, loins and knees, either in direct contact with the skin, or between two gauzes: poultice of raw cabbage leaves, rich in sulfur, cicatrizing and analgesic, poultice of cooked burdock leaves, being careful of hive type reactions.

Les liniments

They are used for local massages of the affected joint:
- Rhus-opodeldoc liniment, for the loins and hips
- Bryonia-opodeldoc liniment, for the knees and small joints.

The Opodeldoc liniment, is an excipient for Rhus tox and Bryonia. It is composed of animal soap, ammonia, camphor and thyme and rosemary essential oils. It greatly calms rheumatic pain and is also used for sprains. It is one of the oldest medications in history.

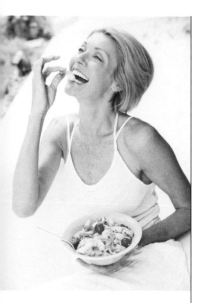

HEALTH PROGRAM FOR YOUR JOINTS

The time has come to change your diet

The diet of a person who suffers from osteoarthritis or arthritis must be adapted to their condition. It is bound to be slightly different from a healthy person's. But the work to be done is absolutely not superhuman.

Your mission: keep your weight under control if you are on the heavy side, create an anti-inflammatory environment, reinforce antioxidant defenses and reinforce your bones and joints. Now, let's look at the details.

Keeping your weight under control

One of the most effective ways of controlling your weight is to only eat for a good reason: when you're hungry. And you can't be hungry all the time. You can have 3 to 5 meals per day, based on your age (5 meals if your are a senior). And no more. To prevent snacking between meals, you need to get rid of hunger pangs. These are greatly dependant on a hormone called insulin, which is produced by the pancreas when you eat and is used to send sugar from food to tissue where it will be used as a source of energy. The more fast release sugars in a meal, the more insulin is secreted. This insulin peak has two consequences: on one hand, it causes blood sugar to drop, which in turn causes a feeling of hunger. On the other hand, it increases the

Oils: saving money

You can find oils called mixed at the supermarket, readily promoted for their beneficial health effects. They are more expensive, but do they keep their promises ? Actually, these oils, like sunflower or corn oils, have a higher omega-6 content. You would save money by using canola oil, perfectly balanced and which is also the cheapest on the market.

synthesis of a chemical brain messenger, adrenalin, which triggers the appetite. In all cases, fast release sugars lead to snacking. To prevent this, researchers first recommend eating less cereal and potatoes (main sources of fast release sugars) than you had before. Do you eat 2 slices of bread at breakfast? Eliminate one. You can compensate for the loss in calories with a little more vegetable protein (soy or quinoa) and fats (up to 40% of your calorie intake). Then, you systematically replace sources of fast release sugars (corn flakes, white bread, pastries, potato chips, French fries, white rice, crackers, candy bars, carbonated soft drinks, candy) with slow release sugars (oats, whole meal bread, pasta, brown rice, almonds, walnuts and hazel nuts).

Creating an anti-inflammatory environment

Fats are the perfect approach for this. The aim is to limit saturated fats (butter and crème fraîche), and introduce monounsaturated olive oil, if you don't use it, and above all to re-establish an equal balance between fats in the omega-6 family and those of the omega-3 family. To do this you need to use canola or nut oils and eliminate sunflower, corn and grape seed oils. You can use olive or canola oil for seasoning and olive oil for cooking. At the same time, you can eat a few walnuts or linseeds each day and fatty fish 2 to 3 times a week (not cooked aggressively: steamed, in a double boiler or poached) and avoid eating tuna too often, due to its mercury contents. You can also take fish oil capsules.

False slow release sugars

Bread and potatoes are often presented as slow release sugars, even by the medical community. Nothing could be further from the truth. These foods have a high glycemic index; this means that they suddenly release their sugar contents during digestion, which leads to a quick rise in blood sugar. These are true fast release sugars. If you can't give up potatoes, try to eat them whole rather than as French fries: they are not as glycemic. The bread with themost beneficial profile is whole, leavened rye bread, not very easy to find.

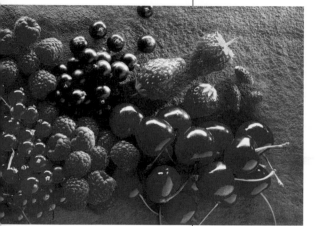

Fruits and vegetables

Your health, and not just that of your joints, depends on antioxidants. So, act accordingly.

More vitamins

Antioxidants are substances which neutralize very aggressive particles called free radicals, responsible for aging. We depend on them every second and even more when the joints are affected, since free radicals are much higher in this case. Researchers are very capable of measuring our ability to neutralize free radicals in our plasma. People who eat more fruit, vegetables and whole foods rich in antioxidants (vitamins C and E, carotenoids and polyphenols) have a higher antioxidant capacity. In these people the aging process in

The limitations of diet

Normally food should supply us with enough antioxidants. However, food studies show that much of the population, even if correctly nourished, does not receive enough. A study on 13,000 people revealed a risk of vitamin C and E deficiency which involves more than one person out of three. The situation is similar for antioxidant minerals. According to a 1991 study, more than 80% of the population does not get the recommended amounts of zinc. A woman needs 50 to 70 micrograms (mcg) of selenium per day. But in reality, food does not supply more than 40 mcg.

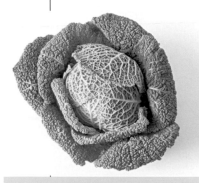

general and that of joint aging are slowed. To do what they do, ideally you'd have to eat 5 to 10 portions of fruits and vegetables daily, if possible rich in antioxidants. This is the case of berries (redcurrants, blackberries, raspberries, strawberries and blueberries), grapes, oranges, tangerines, grapefruit, lemons, plums, dates, pineapples and kiwis. For vegetables higher concentrations are found in red cabbage, bell peppers, parsley, artichokes and spinach. Walnuts are an excellent source of antioxidants.

More phase 2 enzymes

What are they? These enzymes, not well known by the medical community, nevertheless exist in our cells. Their function? To eliminate all the toxic substances in food, like pesticides. But these enzymes also have an antioxidant function, only discovered by researchers at the beginning of the 2000's. Thus these enzymes complete the protection offered by traditional antioxidants such as vitamin C. Their advantage: they can work permanently as long as you regularly eat very special foods which "activate" them. They are found in all crucifer vegetables (*see box*) but also in ginger, carrots, celery, asparagus, green onions, leeks, lettuce and spinach.

Crucifers

The family of the Brassica genus includes 400 members, the best known are: cauliflower, red and white cabbage, Brussel sprouts, Chinese cabbage, borecole, Roman cauliflower, kohlrabi, broccoli, radish, black radish, turnip, rutabaga, horseradish, watercress, canola seed and mustard. "Cabbage was not eaten by the Jews, nor by the Egyptians, Jed Fahey recounted (John Hopkins University, Baltimore, Maryland). On the other hand, it was in the diet of the Greeks and Romans. Cato recommended eating cabbage to prevent chronic diseases. He attributed the existence of his 28 children to it." In the 17th century fermented cabbage embarked on ships since it had been discovered that it prevented scurvy. Currently, crucifers are one of the ten most cultivated plant families in the world.

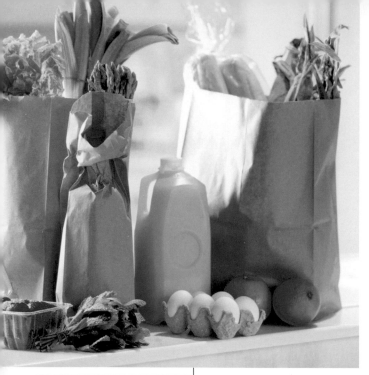

War against weight

VYou need to carefully monitor your weight. You knees and hips suffer from the slightest extra weight. So when you weigh a couple of extra pounds you overload your hips by ten due to a complex mechanical action which destroys the cartilage and causes pain when you walk. So avoid fattening starchy and sugary foods. Use little salt, drink 1 to 1.5 quarts of water per day. Drink wine in moderations and choose very tanniny reds, for example Bordeaux, Californian.

Vegetables against rheumatisms

Certain vegetables can help you fight your rheumatisms. They will be the base of your diet. Slip them into your basket when you're shopping.

The best way to prepare them is to eat them raw in salads (dressed with lemon juice and olive oil) or steamed. You'll benefit from their minerals, vitamins, and the fibers necessary for regulating your intestine and assimilating calcium. You can also put them in the blender to make fresh juice to serve as a cocktail or drink first thing in the morning. A nice glass of carrot juice is excellent from the viewpoint of general drainage. Among all the vegetables you can find at a farmer's market, I'd recommend four: celery, cabbage, tomato and garlic. Rheumatics, get to know all their benefits.

Celery

(Apium graveolens, Umbelliferae family)

They are two types (stalk celery (*dulu* variety) and cele-
riac (*rapaceum* variety). Originally from Italy, these two
celeries appeared late, at the end of the 16th century.
Apium, the wild ancestor of celery, was a sacred plant.
Its original name is Celtic which meant, from an ancient
root "water". There you'll find the relationship between
rheumatism and the humidity which aggravates it. In
the Odyssey, Odysseus took a significant stock with him
for his Mediterranean voyage. Only cultivated celery
should be eaten since the wild variety can be toxic. The
leaves and roots are rich in an aromatic essential oil,
resin, B group vitamins and minerals. It is a great tonic.
Its juice, prepared in a blender is fortifying and anti-
rheumatic. A glass before a meal gives you an appetite
and stimulates digestion. I especially like wine mixed
with celery. Steep 100 g of fresh celery stalks and 100 g
of dried fennel seeds in 1 quart of sweet white wine for
2 days. Shake each day. Filter. Drink one to two glasses
per day. Drink in moderation.

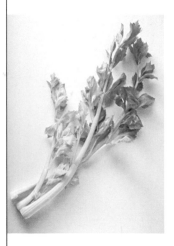

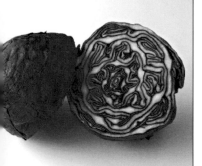

Cabbage: not just in your plate

Poultices of fresh cabbage leaves applied to a painful and deformed joint are also useful. I remember a case of resistant sciatica, worse at night which was remarkably relieved by placing large raw cabbage leaves on the buttock and lumbar spine kept on all night scotch taped to the skin. Painful knees also benefit from these applications.

Cabbage

(*Brassica oleracea, crucifer* family)

Cabbage is a close friend of all phytotherapist doctors. Cultivated for a very long time, popular with the Greeks, Romans and Celts, there is a mass of varieties spread throughout the entire world. Cato the Elder praised it two centuries before Christ and Pliny considered it as the guaranteed means for doing without a doctor, which is not very polite for us. With internal use or as a plaster or poultice, cabbage enjoys a well-deserved popularity. A abbage treatment consists of eating 400 g of cabbage per day, half raw and half cooked. It helps slim, like the famous cabbage soup, loosens the joints and embellishes the skin. My first contact in a medical framework with this vegetable was an elderly woman who, by applying cabbage leaves, had managed to cicatrize a terrible ulcer eating away at her varicose leg. All of the phlebologists in the place were astonished. Cabbage is rich in vitamin C which gives it strong anti-scurvy properties and in vitamin K, which reinforces the bones. Like most crucifers, it contains a sulfur substance which makes it antiseptic and revulsive, but also good for your rheumatisms. For osteoarthritis purposes, it needs to be consumed in a blended fresh juice, one large glass per day, being aware that red cabbage is more active than white cabbage due to the pigments it contains. Lastly, don't forget the benefits of sauerkraut for dieting. Eaten without cured meat, sauerkraut is perfectly easy to digest. As long is it does not contain too much salt, it drains kidneys and joints wonderfully, lowering the uric acid and creatinine levels in the blood.

Tomato

(*Lycopersicum esculentum*, *Solanaceae* family)

The tomato is good for rheumatism even though some unjustly accuse it of causing uric acid to climb. It was the Spaniards who discovered the tomato in America, in Peru and Mexico, where it grows wild, in small scarlet balls. It was introduced to Europe around 1550 but was only grown as an ornamental plant since its toxicity was feared. However, in the Midi of France, it was already popular. Italy attributed it with aphrodisiac virtues. And it was the inhabitants of Marseilles, who mounting an attack against Paris in 1789 brought the Parisians the tomato along with the Marseillaise. It is interesting thanks to its lycopene and antioxidant carotenoid pigments which osteoarthritis sufferers often lack. But it needs to be very ripe. The green tomato is poisonous as are the stalk and its leaves. It contains an alkaloid, solanine, toxic for the central nervous system. The juice of a very red tomato is refreshing and healthy, and eliminates uric acid. Drink one large glass per day. It will protect your cartilage but also your arteries.

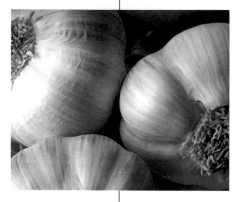

Garlic

(Allium sativum, Alliaceae family)

Garlic, the result of the wild Asian garlic was already cultivated in Palestine 2,000 year before our era. It was popular with the Jews. It can be found, like the onion, depicted on the frescos of Egyptian tombs. The Greeks and Romans devoured large quantities of it. Dioscorides sung its praises. In the Middle Ages, Saint Hildegard and Albertus Magnus made a panacea of it, and the good king Henry IV devoured it with relish. One of my friends, an old doctor in hedge farmland country in the Vendee, treated his rheumatic patients by making them drink a glass of excellent white wine every day where 2 or 3 large garlic cloves had been steeped. It has a rather strong taste but is quite effective, marvelous for your physical shape. Garlic is remarkably diuretic. It doubles the quantity of urine produced. Its spicy flavor and the irritation it causes to the nose and eyes are due to its sulfur compound containing allicin, which is also antiseptic. It is rich in potassium – more than the onion – trace elements, vitamins, iodine and even traces of uranium. Chopped or sliced, it goes well in all your salads. It improves circulation, keeping your joints in good condition.

Herbs

I also attach great importance to "herbs" and "herbes de Provence". I have remarked that those who use these herbs would be better off than others. These herbs are rich in polyphenol molecules, with antioxidant properties, but also terpenes which have the originality of "talking" with our cells, to keep them from undesirably transforming – as brilliantly demonstrated by Dr Michael Sporn from the Dartmouth Medical School (Hanover, New Hampshire). This partly explains the low cancer rates in populations who consume herbs. So season your salads with green onions, savory and tarragon, these are the most effective. Use parsley sparingly, it is too rich in oxalic acid for your kidneys. Spread thyme, oregano and wild thyme on your grilled fish. There is nothing better for your rheumatisms. And in addition, you will neutralize the toxic molecules which often form when cooking proteins.

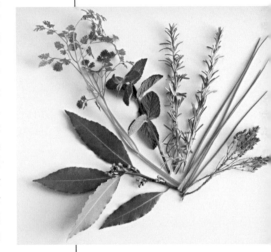

The virtues of vegetables

Many other vegetables are useful for draining the osteoarthritis terrain. You need to know them to incorporate them in your menus as frequently as possible. These vegetables are carrots, lettuce, lamb's lettuce, horseradish, Jerusalem artichoke and salsify. Corn, whose styles, the "awns", are rich in salicylic acid, allow you to prepare excellent herb teas.

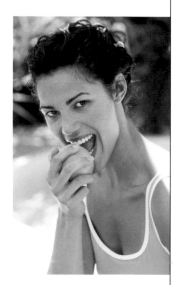

Fruit at your service

Wonderful summer fruit are precious for fighting joint pain and morning stiffness.

There are some that I particularly recommend for my patients, either as part of their daily diet, or as a treatment for a few days. Blueberries, apples, grapes and cherries would be my choices at the market.

Blueberry
(Vaccinium myrtillus)

This is one of the best remedies against rheumatism. This shrub grows wild in northern and eastern Europe as well as in Asia. But it is grown in all of the temperature northern hemisphere. It is the blue colored berries we are interested in. They are rich in vitamins and essential oils which gives them their characteristic scent and flavor and anthocyanic pigments which give them a vascular protection activity. The blueberry leaves are actually diuretic. But it is the berries which are effective for a treatment. Not only do they improve vision bit they have an analgesic and anti-inflammatory action, effectively stimulating the adrenal glands. This action is similar to cortisone without having the toxicity.

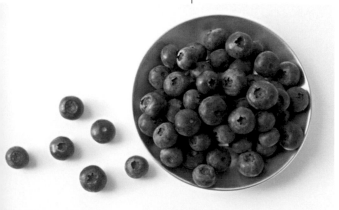

Apple

(Malus communis)

The apple tree is found frequently in our countries: Known from the most ancient of times (don't forget that our mother Eve made our father Adam bite into an apple), our apple tree comes from different hybrids of Asian apple trees where they spread and European apple trees. The apple tree was introduced in the 11th century and its cider, a national drink much loved by William the Conqueror, was from his time. The brut is better than the sweetened type. Very early, the apple was used to fight rheumatisms. Apple tress flourished elsewhere in Virginia where the climate is particularly damp. I highly recommend that my rheumatic patients eat an unpeeled apple at each meal. It will fight your pain and lower cholesterol and uric acid. The apple improves calcium fixation and also fights demineralization and osteoporosis. Moreover, ten days per month, drink 3 cups a day of a tea prepared by letting 50 g of dried and pulverized peels steep in 1 liter of boiling water. Apple peels are excellent against excess uric acid and rheumatic diathesis.

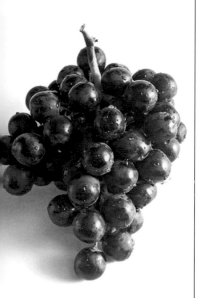

Grape *(Vitis vinifera)*

This is the third fruit to taste. The culture of the vine dates back to the dawn of time. It supposedly originated in Asia Minor, and even millenniums before our era, our ancestors knew how to grow it, and by pressing the grapes and fermenting the juice to obtain wine, a sacred drink par excellence inscribed in our collective unconscious as an archetype. The Greeks introduced the vine to Europe when they founded Marseilles in the 6th B.C. It climbed all along the valley of the Rhone. The Romans then monks ensured its expansion. Currently the limit of vines, after moving very high towards the North, has regressed towards the south stabilizing from Champagne to Hungary with a few exceptions. Fresh grapes contain around 80% water, 15% sugars, proteins and minerals mainly potassium, a diuretic. It is rich in trace elements and vitamins of the B group, and vitamins C and A. With the anthocyanic pigments of its peel, the black grape is an effective protector for our veins and irrigates our cartilage.

A fall treatment

I highly recommend that all of my osteoarthritis patients do a short but effective treatment. To do this, based on your appetite eat two to four pounds per day of good ripe black grapes which you have carefully washed. Chew the seeds and peel well. Do not eat anything else. This detoxifying and diuretic treatment, can be done one more time without any problems at a seven or fifteen day interval. It lowers uric acid, purines, urea and cholesterol. It is indicated for those afflicted with osteoarthritis and gout. You'll see your inflamed joints be relieved of swelling and congestion. Flexibility and easy movements are restored, particularly active on small joints.

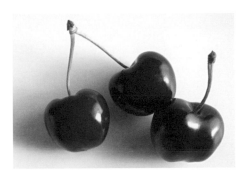

Cherry *(Cerasus vulgaris)*

Nicolas Lemery, the eminent alchemist, considered cherries as "cordials, gastric, aperitifs, appropriate for sweetening the causticness of a bad mood.." It was Dr François-Joseph Cazin who introduced the "cherry stem" tea to therapy, actually the fruit peduncle. This brew, thanks to its high potassium content, is very diuretic. One or two cups a day lowers blood pressure and helps shed pounds. I prescribe it frequently. It helps me avoid chemical diuretics. Lastly, here is a recipe for a very pleasant original drink which is easy to make, healthy and hygienic: Boils 30 g of cherry stems (a large handful) in 1 quart of water. In season pour this boiling brew over 250 g of very ripe cherries cut into pieces (reverchon or coeur de pigeon varieties). Let them sit for 20 minutes, then strain. You'll obtain a delicious beverage to drink chilled, energetically draining your joints. But the period of fresh cherries is short. When the season is over replace them with dry stems mixed with fresh apples cut into pieces.

Other fruits of interest for rheumatics

We'll mention lemons, redcurrants, pears and above all strawberries, unfortunately responsible for numerous allergies. Drinking a glass of juice every day blended from one of these good fruits, selected based on taste, provides excellent benefits for our rheumatic patients. I just finished a terrible rheumatism crisis of a charming elderly woman who could barely walk by prescribing her 2 glasses of pear juice per day.

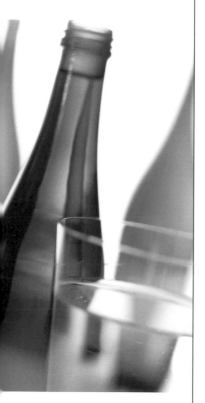

Indispensable minerals

To reinforce your bones and joints you need to eat calcium. But that is not enough.

Definitely calcium

Calcium is necessary for correct constitution of the bony skeleton. Actually, calcium associated with phosphate fixes it on the bones: it guarantees good bone density and thus solidity. Bone metabolism is disturbed in joint diseases. Thus the interest in paying attention to anything that can reinforce it. In addition, calcium associated with vitamin C appears very interesting in treating osteoarthritis. A study published in 2003 found that a daily supplement of one gram of calcium ascorbate (a calcium salt rich in vitamin C) reduces the pain of knee osteoarthritis after just two weeks of treatment. People often look to milk for calcium. But be careful, milk must not be our only source since its proteins sometimes cause allergies and its fats are not good for the arteries. You can eat yogurt, some goat or ewe milk cheeses. Sardines with bones, citrus fruit, almonds, fish and seafood, cabbages, olives, raisins and berries, crucifer vegetables (broccoli,

Premonition

In 1968, the Americans Aaron Wachman and Daniel Bernstein were the first to issue the hypothesis that bone calcium is used by the body to neutralize the excess acid load in the diet. The wrote premonitorily: "It may be interesting to decrease bone loss through a diet which promotes "alkaline ashes". This type of diet places priority on the ingestion of fruits, vegetables, vegetable proteins and a moderate quantity of milk."

Brussel sprouts, borecole and Chinese cabbage) are also good sources of calcium. And, 100 g of Chinese cabbage gives the body more calcium that a glass of milk. Some mineral waters represent a greater intake of calcium if consumed in sufficient quantity: 1.5 to 2 quarts a day.

Acid-base balance

The diet supplies hydrogen and sulfate (acids) or bicarbonate (bases) ions. Based on whether the former predominate or not, the blood is more or less acid. When it is too acid, the body draws calcium from the bone to neutralize the excess acidity. The diet in effect since the Neolithic, rich in cereals, dairy products, salt and sugar is highly acidic. On the other hand a diet rich in vegetables, which adds potassium (a base load) creates immunity to acidity and allows better bone density. Thus it is important to create immunity from acidosis. This is especially the case of people who suffer from joint inflammation. A study showed that inflammation accompanies acidosis in the joints. Actually, as the disease progresses the more the acid-base balance is disturbed. The acid-base balance can be re-established by eating less cereal, dairy products, salt and sugar and a little more fruit and vegetables, dried fruit and nuts. You can also complete this with potassium bicarbonate capsules sold in drugstores.

What to do if calcium is not retained?

The needs of the body: the higher they are (growth, pregnancy or nursing) the more dietary calcium is retained; The dose: you assimilate calcium better when the doses are broken up during the day; Vitamins D and K improve the absorption and retention of calcium; Potassium salts, fruits and vegetables add a sharp base load which limits bone calcium losses; Physical exercise: that which exerts a physical stress on the bone (bodybuilding and dancing) reduce the loss of calcium; tobacco, caffeine, alcohol, salt, excess animal proteins, certain medications (corticosteroids) contribute to calcium loss.

A diet to correct acidosis

An alkaline diet, which you can start today. Here are the main principles.

Food type	To eat	To avoid
Meats	Poultry (chicken, duck, guinea fowl, turkey, duck... without the skin), beef and lamb. Eat lean cuts.	Fatty cuts Industrial packaged cured meats.
Seafood	All fish, in particular herring, salmon; oysters.	Canned fish in oil. Fish eggs. Breaded or fried fish. Smoked fish. Frozen fish gratin.
Eggs	Hard boiled, fried, soft boiled, scrambled and omelets.	Industrial omelets. Eggs in aspic.
Vegetables and fruit	All fresh or frozen vegetables. All fresh fruit. Legumes: peas, white or red beans, broad beans and soy beans. Almonds, hazelnuts	Canned vegetables, packaged or canned soups. Canned fruit in syrup. Freeze-dried mashed potatoes, chips. Grilled and salted dried fruit (used for cocktails).
Cereal	Whole meal bread made from different grains. Brown rice, wild rice, basmati rice.	White bread, sandwich loaf, cookies. Fast cooking white rice, frozen cooked rice.

Food type	To eat	To avoid
Cereal *(continued)*	Whole meal pasta Müesli without sugar, oat-meal.	Fast cooking pasta. Corn flakes and all puffed and sugary breakfast cereals Sugary industrial pastries and cookies. Crackers. Pizza, quiches and savory pies.
Dairy products	Plain yogurt, fresh cheese (to be eaten sparingly)	Industrial cheeses. Sugary yogurts and other milk-based desserts. Chocolate milk.
Fatty and oily materials, seasonings and condiments	Olive, canola, walnut and soy oil Canola margarine. Unsalted peanuts, maca-damia nuts and pista-chios. Garlic, onion, shallot, parsley, basil, tarragon, green onion, thyme, rose-mary, bay leaf, etc.	Salted butter and fresh cream. Solid grease for frying. Bouillon cubes, packaged stocks for sauce, fish sauce, Kikkoman soy sauce (Teriyaki) Mustard, ketchup. Bottled dressing. Cornichons.
Beverages	Uncarbonated mineral water rich in calcium and magnesium Alkaline carbonated mine-ral water. Fresh fruit juice or 100% pure juice with no added sugar. Herb teas. Wine (1 to 2 glasses per day).	Tomato juice. Sodas. **With moderation:** alcohol, coffee, tea.

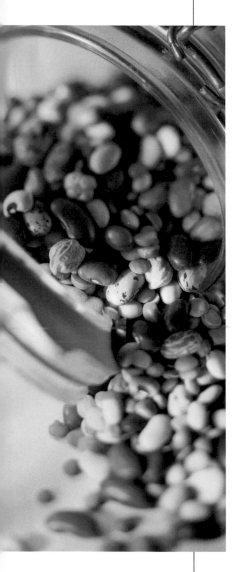

An alkaline diet in practice

In detail, food group by food group, the recommendations for an alkaline diet.

A rule to remember: for each part of acid food (offal, meat, dairy products, cereals, certain dried legumes and certain nuts) eat two parts alkaline food (fruit, vegetables, certain carbonated mineral waters).

Fruits, vegetables and legumes: at least seven portions per day

Fruit and vegetables should be the main part of your diet, both in volume and weight. All fruits and vegetables are good to eat, at the rate of at least seven portions per day. Fruit juice can replace a portion of fruit but only once a day. A part of soup counts for a portion of vegetables as long as it is homemade and not too salty. Buy fruits and vegetables in season. Legumes can be eaten at a rate of ate least three portions per week. Legumes are acid but moderately so. This is especially true for tofu (soy), chick peas and lentils. However, soy milk, green beans and peas are not very acid.

Fat materials and nuts two to four portions per day

There are no special remarks about added fats, as long as they comply with the correct balance between fatty acids: canola and olive oil and canola margarine for seasoning, olive oil for cooking, goose fat if needed. It is preferable to buy virgin oils. Butter is to be used sparingly because it contains saturated fats and is slightly acid. Nuts are included in this group. The most acid nuts are Brazil nuts, followed by cashews. The least acid are pecans.

Cereals: zero to six portion per day

Cereals on the whole are acid. This is particularly true for breakfast cereals, like Special K or All Bran, pizzas, rice crackers, crepes, pastries, pound cake and ladyfingers. Bread is moderately acid, just like rice. Chocolate sandwich cookies, fruit filled cookies, brown rice, wild rice, spice cake and spaghetti are not very acid. To correct significant acidosis you can selectively or permanently eliminate cereals, as is the case in a Paleolithic diets. If you eat them, you should choose fairly unprocessed cereals, whole meal bread with grains and leavened, brown rice and whole or semi-whole meal pasta.

A return to health

For thousands of years humans essentially ate game (around 35% of calories) and wild plants (leaves, roots and berries) (around 65% of calories). Professor Anthony Sebastian, a professor of medicine at the University of California, San Francisco, evaluated the acid load on the model of prehistoric diet, i.e. the net acid production (NAP) and compared it to that of of modern diets. From an average of - 88 mEq/day, meaning a very alkaline diet more than 10,000 years ago we have passed to an average of +48 mEq/day, meaning a highly acid diet. So we now find ourselves in a context completely the opposite of the first humans. And from a genetic viewpoint, we are no different from them. To function correctly, our organism needs to be in a slightly base environment to be in good health. We need to return to an alkaline diet.

Cured meats: zero to three portion per week

It is not a good idea to eat too many cured meats, since the increase the risk of digestive cancer due to the nitrites they contain. Sausage, blood sausage, mortadella, foie gras, potted meats are moderately acid. Ham and salami are a little more.

Fish, shellfishes, shells: three portions a week

Like all animal proteins, fish, crustaceans and shellfish are acid, but there are differences. Fish and seafood which should be eaten in moderation include canned salmon, salted cod, fish eggs, canned tuna in oil, carp, cuttlefish, fresh red tuna (cooked), swordfish, canned sardines in oil, white tuna in oil, salmon, surimi, raw red tuna, tuna in water and pike. Seafood which is less acid, in order from less acid to more acid are oysters (especially with lemon!), grouper, pickled herring, wild salmon, lobster, turbot, scallops, octopus, fresh albacore tuna (cooked), whiting, cod, shrimp, mullet, rainbow trout, squid and mackerel.

Dairy products: zero to two per day

The most acid dairy products are cheeses, and among these parmesan, fondue, Swiss cheese, comté, gruyere, raclette, morbier, and goat cheese. A little less acid – and thus to give priority to if you love cheese – munster, cantal, mozzarella, Roquefort and saint-nectaire. Even less acid: camembert, blue cheese, feta, reblochon, brie and coulommiers. fresh cheese, yogurt and milk are moderately or slightly acid.

French fries, candy, industrial cakes, pastries, sodas, grilled salted nuts: zero to three portions per week

These foods are to be eaten sparingly, for reasons which are often different from the acid base balance: they increase blood sugar or introduce toxic compounds (transfat, products of advanced glycation).

Water: 1.5 to 2 quarts a day

You can drink tap water but it is better if you get information from your water board on the frequency and results of analyses made on the water quality, in particular on the level of nitrates and pesticides. If you opt for bottled water, it is advisable to drink at least half of an alkaline water. These is usually carbonated water. To select an alkaline water, read the labels and look for a water whose level of bicarbonates is around 1,000 mg/l (at least) with a low chloride quantity (less than 50 mg/l) and low fluorine quantity (less than 4 mg/l).

How can I eat less salt?

A crucial part of the alkaline diet: less salt. Anyone is capable of decreasing their salt intake.

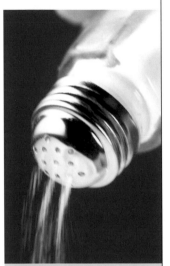

Where is the salt hidden?

– Salt naturally contained in foods: 10%
- Salt added when cooking or at the table: 15%
- Salt added during industrial processing: 75 %

Reducing salt consumption is not that easy, since it is not the salt shaker on the table that is the problem, but the "hidden" salt contained in industrial foods. This represents between 70 and 80% of the salt we absorb. An excellent preservative, taste enhancer, it improves the flavor and appearance of food. In fact, it is everywhere, even where you wouldn't expect it: chocolate, biscuits, yogurt, milk-based desserts, sodas, etc. The main salt-carrying foods are bread and bakery products, cured meats, soups, cheeses, prepared foods, pizzas, quiches and savory tarts, sandwiches, pastries, seafood products, meats and poultry, condiments and sauces. To eat less salt, common sense dictates to consume fewer industrial products rich in salt, and to give priority to fresh products, cooked at home and to go lightly with the salt shaker.

Some tips for reducing your salt intake

• Get rid of the habit of adding salt to everything you eat. Initially, food will seem bland, but your taste buds will get used to it. You'll rediscover the real taste of foods; the pleasure of eating will be the order of the day. The more you do this, the more you will spontaneously

What are our sodium needs?

Theoretically, our physiological needs are met with 2 g of salt per day, i.e. 800 mg of sodium. In France and the United States, healthcare authorities agree to a daily ration of 2.4 g of sodium (i.e. 6 g of salt per day).

turn down foods which are too salty. You'll only need to follow your instincts.

The surprises of canned foods

	Potassium	Sodium
Raw string beans (100 g)	243 mg	4 mg
Cooked string beans (100 g)	240 mg	3 mg
Canned string beans (100 g)	107 mg	307 mg

• Replaces salt with other condiments: garlic, parsley, celery, onion, thyme, herbes de Provence and pepper. On the other hand, avoid mustard (very high in salt), as well as many other industrial condiments (beef or chicken bouillon cubes, ready-made sauces, ketchup, bottled dressings). Use a "salt" rich in potassium.

Recommendations in the United States

The American Institute of Medicine in February 2004 proposed an optimal intake of around 1.5 g of sodium and 2.3 g of chloride per day; i.e. a total of 3.8 g of salt, and recommended not to eat more than 5.8 g.

• Limit cured meats, ready-cooked meals, canned foods, smoked fish, potato chips, crackers and roasted, salted salted nuts.

• Rinse canned vegetables to get rid of as much salt as possible.

• Avoid putting salt in the water when you cook pasta, rice or vegetables.

• Do not let your children get used to eating too much salt, since eating habits acquired as a child are hard to change as an adult

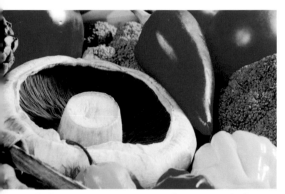

Potassium for your cells

Fruits and vegetables are our main source of potassium. And we should return to giving them priority.

What are our potassium needs?

Unlike vitamins, there is no recommended nutritional amount for potassium. However, faced with the importance of health problems due to too much salt consumption and industrial foods to the detriment of fresh foods, the American Institute of Medicine proposed in February 2004 to take "at least" 4.7 g of potassium per day *(see the table below)*.

Adequate potassium intake

	Age	Men (g/d)	Women (g/d)
Infants	0 to 6 month	0,4	0,4
	7 to 12 month	0,7	0,7
Children	1 to 3 years	3,0	3,0
	4 to 8 years	3,8	3,8
	9 to 13 years	4,5	4,5
Adolescents	14 to 18 years	4,7	4,7
Adults	19 years and older	4,7	4,7
Pregant women	14 to 50 years	-	4,7
Nursing women	14 to 50 years	-	5,1

Where can you find potassium?

There are numerous and varied food sources, since the mineral is the major constituent of plants and animal cells (see table). Even if meat, dairy products and cereals actually contain potassium, overall these foods acidify the body. So it is better to increase the consumption of vegetables.

• Unlimited fruits and vegetables: ideally three to five portions of fruit and four to six portions of vegetables per day. The best sources of potassium (per 100 kcal) are leafy green vegetables (spinach and lettuce), tomato, cucumber, zucchini, eggplant, bell peppers and tubers (carrots, radish and turnips).

• Rediscover almonds, hazel nuts and other nuts. Rich in fiber, they contain good fatty acids (unsaturated fatty acids) and are an excellent source of potassium.

• Consider fruit more often for your light meals or, for the recalcitrant, fruit juice, even if it is not as rich in potassium (take very ripe fruit, centrifuge it and drink it right away). When buying juice, get 100% fruit juice with no added sugar.

Potassium contents (mg/100 g)

Food	mg	Food	mg
Fats	0	Fresh avocado	522
Sugar	0	Fresh spinach	529
Eggs	128	Baked potato	536
White bread	132	Raw black radish	554
Milk	150	Chervil	600
Raspberry, blackberry, peach	220	Date	670
Kiwi, cherry, redcurrant, grape	280	Walnut	690
Whole meal bread	350	Dried lentils	700
Artichoke	350	Roasted peanuts	710
Beef	370	Almond	800
Banana, apricot, coconut	380	Prune	950
Pork	390	Dried banana	1,150
Chocolate	400	Dry white beans	1,450
Fish	400	Dried apricot	1,520
Mushroom	420	Powdered cocoa	1,920
Turkey	490	Red pepper	2,000
Veal	500		

Potassium in salt or gel capsules

If you have a hard time satisfying the rule of seven portions of fruits and vegetables per day, there are potassium supplements which can be used to make up these amounts.

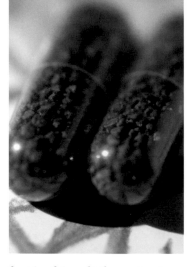

Swap your table salt for potassium salt

Potassium salt is a dietetic salt found in drugstores; it is used like a normal salt. Rich in potassium (30%), it contains very little sodium (8%) while maintaining the salty taste of traditional salt. It is important to note that in this salt the potassium is linked to bicarbonate, the form in which it is found in vegetables and not to chloride (not much present in fruits and vegetables).

Potassium supplements

When the diet does not contain adequate quantities of potassium, you can use supplements. Potassium gel capsules are available at the drugstore in bicarbonate form. The recommended dosage is 2 to 4 gel capsules per day. For people in good health, a potassium dietary intake above the recommended nutritional amount is not dangerous since the excess potassium is simply eliminated in the urine.
Thus the supplements are harmless.

Who should not take a supplement?

People who suffer from hyperkalemia. People who take potassium retaining diuretics, angiotensin-converting enzyme inhibitors or digitalis glycosides. Generally, people with heart disease, diabetics, kidney disease, pregnant and nursing women should ask their doctor for advice before taking a potassium supplement.

Monitor your magnesium

To correct a potassium deficiency, it is indispensable to have a satisfactory magnesium level. The cells cannot retain potassium without magnesium.

Magnesium is the second intercellular cation in terms of importance. Like potassium, it is abundant in all vegetables. Magnesium is an alkalizing mineral which contributes to restoring the acid-base balance.

Magnesium deficiencies are frequent

Magnesium comes entirely from our food. But current diets are far from covering our needs. According to a Suvimax study conducted on 5,000 people, 77% of women and 72% of men have magnesium quantities less than the daily recommended amounts (recommended nutritional amount: adult women: 360 mg, adult men: 420 mg). There are several reasons for the deficiencies. Current diets contains many processed foods to the detriment of vegetable products. In addition, stress generates physiological mechanisms which consume a lot of magnesium.

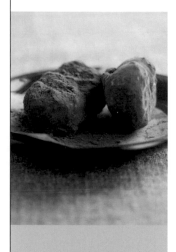

Food sources of magnesium

- Fruits and vegetables (almonds win the prize: 275 mg of magnesium per 100 g).
- Chocolate: more than 300 mg per 100 g.
- Some mineral waters

Magnesium as a food supplement

Gel capsules of magnesium carbonate or dolomite gel capsules can be found in drugstores (double carbonate of calcium and magnesium).

165

Sports

Sports are not the enemy of osteoarthritis, far from it! It is still indispensable to exercise when you have osteoarthritis...but in moderation!

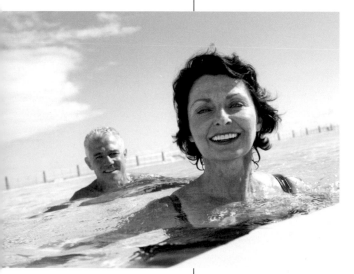

Sports are important throughout life and osteoarthritis should not keep you from pursuing a physical activity. It is absolutely imperative to continue to walk every day, to force yourself to exercise, even if your joints are painful. It just involves adapting the intensity and duration of the effort to the condition of your joints. Sports are necessary: they make it possible to preserve correct mobility of affected joints and keep muscles and the joints which surround the joint strong. Physical activity also stimulates vascularization of the tissues around the joint and thus cartilage synthesis.

Do athletes have more osteoarthritis?

In young people sports which subject the joints to strong pressure and twisting like skiing can promote osteoarthritis of the knee or hip. It is primarily joint traumas due to sports that result in a predisposition to the disease. Other sports like running or soccer may promote osteoarthritis only if they are practiced intensively, in competition for many years.

Move... but be gentle with your joints

Choose a sport which does not strain your joints too much. Tennis games and bike rides are over! It is better to turn to swimming and gymnastics in the pool that let you work your joints gently. Water decreases the weight the joints need to support and its resistance works the muscles more or less based on the speed of the movements. These activities are particularly recommended for people who are overweight. "Dry" gymnastics are also useful.

Older people too!

In order to precisely assess the benefits of sports on osteoarthritis, American researchers studied 439 people aged 60 or over for 18 months. They all suffered from osteoarthritis of the knee at a stage which hampered their freedom of movement. The participants did resistance exercises (such as lifting weights) and sports (walking, swimming and gym). At the end of the study all the participants reported suffering less, and had less difficulty lifting and carrying loads. They walked faster and took less time to go up and down stairs or get out of their car. According to the American team, regular physical activity should be prescribed, and given the same weight as medications, as part of the treatment of osteoarthritis.

Sports to live a long life

Numerous studies have demonstrated that older people who practice a physical activity several times a week have a better mineral bone density than those who are inactive- Bodybuilding exercises 3 times a week for 6 months have let elderly men and women from age 60 to 83 to reinforce their hip bone density.

Saving your back and joints

When you have osteoarthritis and even before it starts, you need to be careful to protect your joints by adopting appropriate movements.

It is during daily life and for your entire life that your uselessly tire your joints. Standing up, bending over, sitting or carrying packages....you do these things every day, but do you do them right? Here are some tips for saving your joints. Good habits to make ...and, more importantly, maintain!

Generally, everyone should avoid:
* tiring positions for long periods of time. If you need to remain standing or sitting for many hours in a row, take short breaks to walk, you should stretch and relax your muscles at least every two hours;
* sudden movements and twisting which put the bones out of alignment related to the joint. For example, twisting of the spine uselessly wears the vertebra joints. Turn around completely to see things going on behind you.

Standing

The spine needs to stay in its natural curve as much as possible. Thus it is necessary to stand up straight, without excessively arching your back nor bending the top part of your back. If you need to stand for a long time,

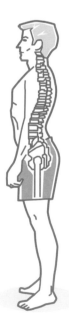
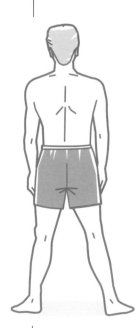

bend your legs a bit and open your feet towards the outside to divide the weight on each side..

Sitting

Always sit completely back in the chair. The back supports your back and keeps you from slouching. The arms are supported on the arm rests. The television needs to be straight ahead and at the height of the eyes. At work, your feet should be lifted and your seat adjusted to the right height for your desk.

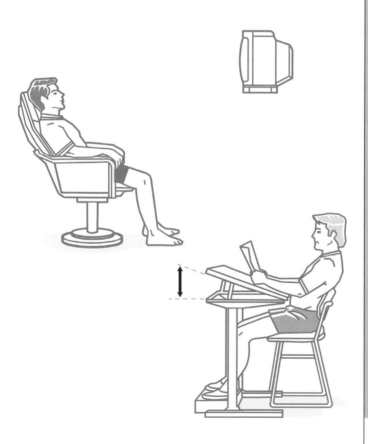

Tai chi, a source of well-being

An American study demonstrated that practicing tai chi daily relieves the pain of osteoarthritis! This martial art, completely gentle, involves making movements which improve blood circulation and reinforce the tissue near the joints. It is thanks to these effects that the pain is relieved. According to an American study, people aged 68 to 87 complain less about the pain of their osteoarthritis after 10 weeks of working out. In addition, and we often forget the importance of mood in pain management, tai chi letsyou gain self-control, of your breathing and inner energy. It also boosts morale. So practice as much as you want!

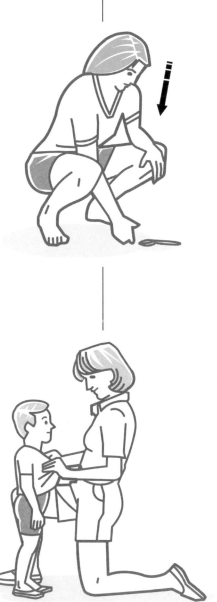

Bending down

Always bend your knees and do not strain your spine. To pick up an object, you can bend both knees to get down to the ground or slightly bend one knee and use your other leg for balance using one hand for support, for example on a table. To take care of children, put one knee on the floor, to keep your back straight instead of leaning forward.

Lifting and carrying packages

For everyday things, divide the bags on each side of the body. For heavy loads: take the object from the back between your legs then stand up keeping your back straight to balance and support the heavy object against your thigh. Always carry loads very close to your body.

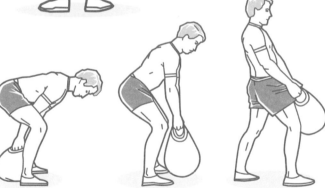

A good comfortable bed?

Try to sleep in a bed which is not too soft, and which does not sink too much under the weight of your body. Change your bedding every 10 years. Mattresses in wool should be avoided. Large pillows should also be avoided as well as thick bolsters: sleeping with the head too far forward is one of the main causes of cervical pain and stiffness. One the other hand, to read laying down the pillow should be under your shoulders and support your nape and upper back. Avoid laying down and getting up abruptly. Support yourself on your legs and arms so that you don't just put stress on your spine.

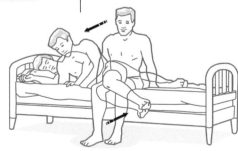

171

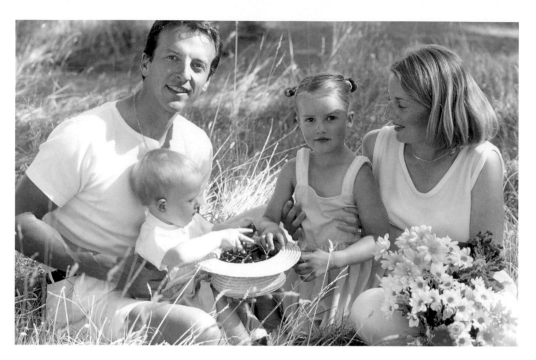

AND TO CONCLUDE WITH A
FLOURISH OF PLANTS

Aging well and staying alert despite the years is an exciting program. You don't need to be a millionaire or head of State to do this. A little bit of security that our society gives to most of us, calculated physical exercise, a good diet, a careful and moderate usage of the medicinal herbs will help you to stay in shape and enjoy life.

Thus plants can effectively help you to refind joint comfort and youth. Treating yourself with plants, finding in the thousands of plant species which surround us those capable of giving us well-being is a desire we all have.

Nature is around us and we have a desire within us to immerse ourselves in it. This craving is tinged with great nostalgia among unhappy city dwellers who live and work in the inferno of concrete and asphalt. A small house with green shutters overlooking a small yard or over a large meadow filled with flowers is the security of a peaceful happiness we all want. We all dream of that path to take the time to exist. The sound of cicada and crickets is much more pleasant than the din of cars and motorcycles. Happiness is in the meadow.

But getting up early in the morning, going out to look for medicinal herbs, picking them still embellished with the rosy morning light full of sunny energy brings immeasurable joy as long as you know a bit of practical botany or you get advice from someone with expertise, for example your druggist, who has studied phytotherapy in-depth.

Drying the plant you have picked will add fragrance to your house, preparing your own teas, poultices and medicinal oils will bring an ineffable pleasure which will in turn activate the beneficial effects of your herbal tea and your liniment.

Ah, that wonderful thyme picked in the neighboring scrubland and the cup of it you drink after breakfast or dinner, how it will drain your bladder, how it will make you digest well, how it will loosen up your joints!

This vision of paradise is a bit like being in Adam and Eve's condition under the apple tree but unfortunately cannot be realized by everyone. So you should know that your druggist can find you gel capsules, single or mixed herb teas, drinkable ampoules which let you satisfy your legitimate desire to return to nature..

Natural does not mean friendly

Nature is not always friendly. A storm, in essence a natural phenomenon, can kill you with lightening. You need to protect yourself from the cold and rain. Natural forces identified by Hippocrates – we are all carriers – are sometimes insufficient for healing us, or for example, during a high fever, may exceed their goal and be life threatening.

Response to eminent scientists

Some scientists who are too full of scientism turn up there noses over these medicinal herbs which they find too simple. I hear them exclaim, outraged: "Here, at a time when science, our science, has discovered antibiotics, synthetic hormones, tranquillizers, anti-depressants, anti-inflammatory drugs, your want to make due by treating with a modest daisy or a simple piece of willow bark? We have extracted the active ingredient from each plant worthy of interest. We have modified it to make it even more active and you want to go back to it! Iconoclast!"

These eminent scholars are both right and wrong

They are wrong because the entire plant represents a "totum", that is a plant entity where the active ingredient's action is supported, softened, enhanced and regulated by the presence of other compounds such as tannins which slow down the absorption of minerals, trace elements which make it more dynamic, pigments which broaden the action. A great, very simple example of this different action of the plant taken as a whole compared to its isolated ingredients is the eucalyptus, an impressive tree whose leaves possess, thanks to an essential oil, balsamic and disinfecting benefits for the bronchial tubes.

But it also has an interesting hypoglycemic action. It is capable of lowering the blood sugar level when it has increased. For this purpose, I use it when treating type 2 diabetes which men and women often suffer from around age fifty from being over-nourished. However, when you analyze eucalyptus and test each of its cons-

Self-medication with plants: use good sense

Treating yourself with medicinal herbs requires using good sense above all. You can only treat complaints which are more of a problem than a real disease: old joint or back pains, digestion, stomach or intestinal problems, a slow bowel, a lack of tone, nervousness and poor circulation, moreover these represent most of the complaints which bother the existence of our fellow creatures. But for a certain, serious disease, your doctor's advice and the use of modern medications is indispensable. In this case plants can only play a supporting role and in this case our scientists are completely right. A serious disease is not treated with plants – or at least not with plants alone.

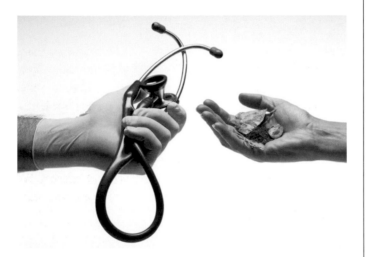

tituents, you notice that taken individually, they don't possess any action on blood sugar. It is all of these ingredients, the plant totum, and only this totum, which is active.

Another example of this is digitalis, whose cardioactive properties we are well aware of. An active ingredient is extracted known by the name crystallized digitalin, or even, with a variation, as digoxin. These hetersidic substances have a very regular, well dosed action. But their serious problem is to cause a loss of blood potassium, an indispensable substance for heartbeat regularity. Thus in our long-term treatments with digitalin, it is necessary to regularly check this blood potassium, kaliemia, and to add to the treatment if the kaliemia

decreases. However, the leaf of the digitalis, and thus the powder prepared from this leaf, contains precisely that quantity of potassium salt necessary for the regularity of this cardioactive action.

Toxic digitalis

My comments about digitalis should not lead you, if you have a heart condition, to pick it yourself and to make herbal tea with it. This is very dangerous and can even be fatal. Digitalis is a strong poison and can only be prescribed by a doctor after several tests.

Plants:
a precious gift

Medicinal plants remain a precious gift of the divinity which guides us or controls us by chance.

Proof of this is the care the World Health Organization takes to check all of the elements which can be contributed by local phytotherapy with the greatest attention. These include the smiling secrets of the old grandmother roosting in a hollow, the unquestionably more fearful secrets of the African witch doctor or traditional Buddhist monk. Thus, the rose periwinkle made its entrance into our therapeutic arsenal against blood cancer. Plants possess their magic which often results in scientific discovery. Having started this phytotherapy bible with stories of my youth, I won't end it without telling you a personal anecdote. It also reinforced my vocation to treat with the "simplicity" of medicinal plants..

Phytotherapy elected by a show of hands

Ages ago, at a time when I was actively involved in politics, I had the chance to follow an important government leader during his electoral campaign. Obviously, I won't say anything more about the person in question. I was part of his team, his staff! Moreover, my medical skills were appreciated. We traveled from city to towns, holding meetings after meetings.

One morning, we were all at breakfast and my politician appeared tired, his features tight and in a bad mood.

The gout he had been harboring for years and for which he had been traditionally treated had irritated his foot all night. Worse, he whispered into my doctor's ear, he had n't urinated all night. He had the impression that his kid neys were blocked, and anxiously wondered if he could continue his campaign. Did I have a quick solution?

The answer was simple. Rather than using just any chemical diuretic which, prescribed without a preliminary exam, would have unquestionably worsen things, I went to the big drugstore in the town. There I bought some solidago herb tea, a type of birch and then had the great man drink two mugs for breakfast.

The next stop was another 120 miles, all in an official car mind you. We had to stop twenty times, meaning every six miles, so that this eminent figure could relieve his bladder on the side of the road. Each time he returned, his face lit up with a big smile, he thanked me for the godsend of this birch which he compared to a magic wand. He drank up the rest of his stock. He had no more problems and was elected, standing on his head I would dare to say.

You'll see what still needs to be done. Plants lead to everything and more importantly will relieve your rheumatisms.

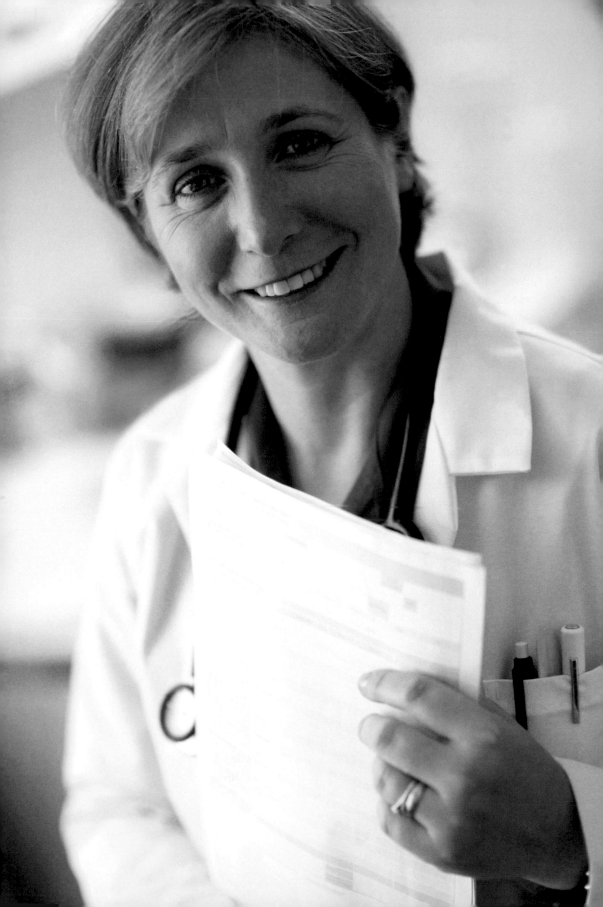

OSTEOARTHRITIS: ACCEPTED IDEAS...

The disease, a source of the unknown and uncertainties, carries with it many preconceived ideas. Our culture, a personal experience or that of a close friend or relative, plenty of elements interfere with our perception of the disease and they vision we have of it. Well here are some elements that will help you separate false from true.

Anti-inflammatory drugs do more harm than good

False! Certainly they cause some significant problems. Heartburn and stomach aches can moderately alter the quality of life. However, it is best to put things into perspective. Serious complications are rare. If you carefully weigh the pros and cons, you'll see that the therapeutic benefits outweigh the side effects..

Plants can cure everything

False. You can't ask plants to do the impossible! They cannot cure certain serious diseases like AIDS, cancer and others. However, they can be used to treat many common complaints and are a precious aid in supporting treatment of certain problems caused by the disease or treatments..

Plants are less effective than chemical medications

True and false... Actually, they do not act in the same way. A plant generally contains numerous active ingredients which can be used for overall treatment of the patient. Chemical medications concentrate one active

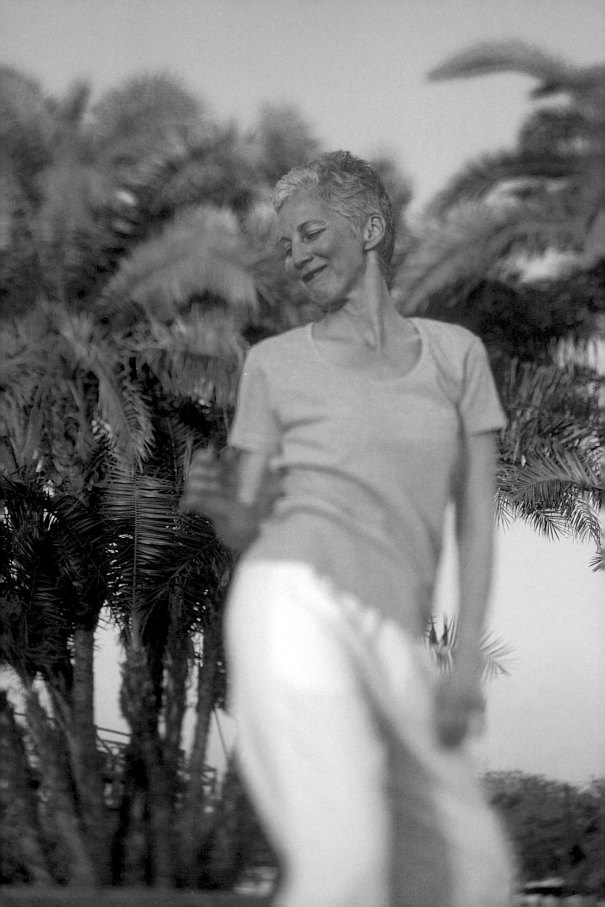

ingredient with the goal of a fast, clear and targeted action. However, it is important to know that many of our modern medications come from plants and very often contain plant extracts or modified vegetable molecules. It is actually within plants that researchers find active substances. For example, digitalin, a treatment for heart failure comes from digitalis, a lively plant which blooms in our forests during the summer.

Osteoarthritis cannot be cured

True. If you stick to precise definitions. The term "cure" indicates that the disease is eradicated from the body where it was running wild. Osteoarthritis is an aging of the joint which cannot be completely eliminated. Treatments make it possible to simply slow down its evolution or to relieve the symptoms.

To decrease pain, it is a good idea to go to bed

True. Actually, your bed is very important for daily "management" of osteoarthritis. By avoiding mattresses which are too soft and sleeping with a pillow, your sleep will be improved. But you also need to be careful to get out of bed correctly: first put your feet on the ground, and once well supported, lift your back keeping it straight.

Pain is a fatality

False. Certainly not! Many people think that it is "normal" to suffer after a certain age: of course not. Pain is an anomaly of functioning. If you need to accept the fact of aging and to no longer be in the same shape as before, you can't forget that there are ways of relieving pain. Knowledge progresses each day and treatments are more and more effective. So, accepting pain to fight against it, that is fine, but resigning yourself to suffering and calling it normal, is not!

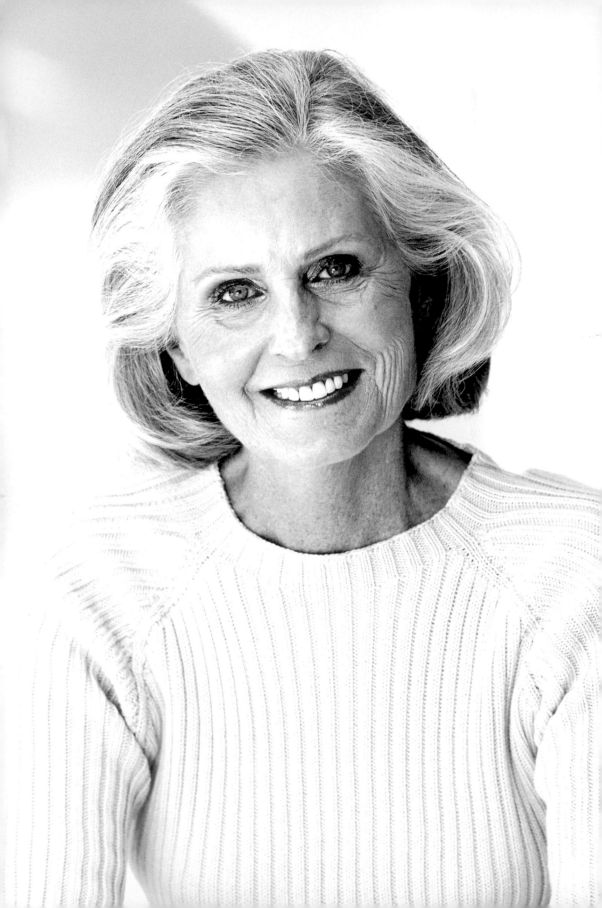

OSTEOARTHRITIS: ANSWERS TO YOUR QUESTIONS

You hear more and more about "chondrocalcinosis". What is it?

This is the second "microcrystalline arthritis" after gout. However, it is undervalued. More and more frequent as one ages, 6% of the population between age 60 and 70 is effected. And up to 50 % over age 90! It is due to deposits of calcium phosphate. Most often, the cause is not found and it can be associated with gout or poor thyroid functioning. In the most common form, it manifests with chronic joint pain. Treatment involves giving anti-inflammatory drugs or injecting corticosteroids in the joint if anti-inflammatory drugs are contraindicated.

Is a cane necessary?

Most people who suffer from osteoarthritis do not need any technical aid. But some elderly people may benefit from one. Canes, tools for getting things on shelves, booster seats for toilets, and support bars on the walls can considerably improve autonomy. You shouldn't hesitate to ask for them when you feel they'd be useful for improving everyday life. An apartment or house can also be fitted. You doctor is in the best position to give you advice.

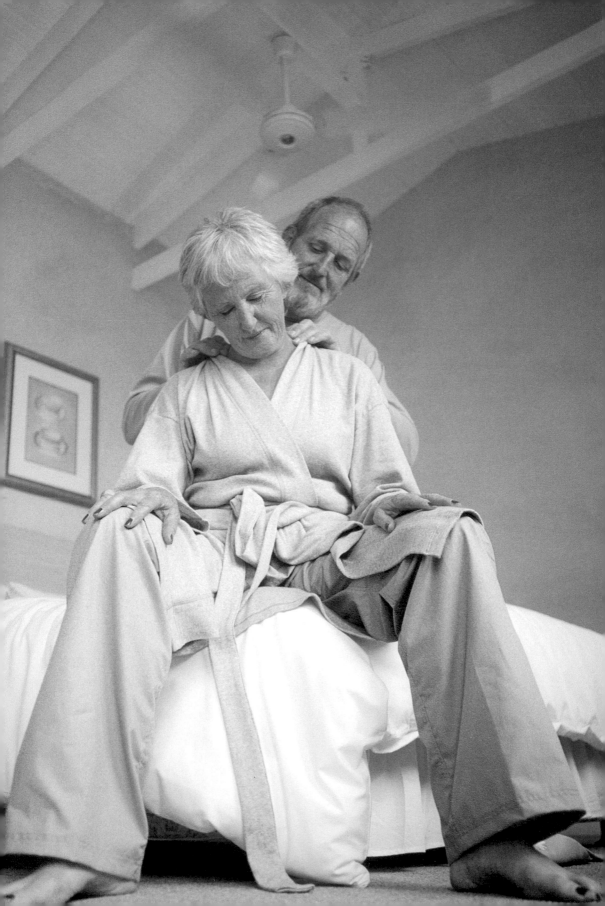

What a joint lavage?

The aim of a joint lavage is to clean out the joint from cartilage debris and residue of inflammation which causes inflammation. To do this the doctor inserts a sterile saline solution into the joint cavity then drains it by suctioning. The operation is performed under a local anesthetic. Done before an injection, a joint lavage increases it effectiveness.

Is rest absolutely necessary?

It is indispensable to take it easy for a few minutes every day, no matter what the stage of osteoarthritis. Resting is not synonymous with doing nothing or lying down. It may also be wearing a splint, resting a painful joint, changing position or activity, and decreasing pressure on the joints..

Is relaxing part of the treatment?

Yes, learning to relax is highly advisable. An indispensable complement to rest and exercise, relaxation lowers the level of stress. And, above all, it increases the effectiveness of times of rest.

GLOSSARY

URIC ACID: acid produced by the break down of nucleic acids (DNA and RNA) of the body and by digestion of foods rich in nucleic acids (liver, calf sweetbreads, certain fish and poultry).

DNA (DEOXYRIBONUCLEIC ACID): molecule which contains the information necessary for the development and functioning of a living being. It is the support for genetic material. It is the main constituent of chromosomes.

ANEMIA: decrease of the quantity of hemoglobin in the blood.

ANTIOXIDANT: substance which protects against free radicals produced by the body during oxidation reactions.

CAROTENOIDS: pigments present in yellow-orange or red-purple vegetables which protects them against being burned by the sun. Carotenoids have antioxidant properties.

CHONDROCYTES: builder cells which ensure cartilage renewal.

CORTICOIDS (CORTICOSTEROID): hormones naturally secreted by the body. The term also refers to medications with chemically produced hormones to use their anti-inflammatory properties.

ESTROGENS: female sexual hormones.

IMMUNITY: all of the mechanisms which protect the body.

INFLAMMATION: localized reaction in a tissue, following an aggression. It manifests with reddening, heat, swelling and pain.

INSULIN: hormone secreted by the pancreas used for the cells to absorb blood sugar.

SYNOVIAL FLUID: fluid present in the joint which serves to lubricate in order to help sliding of the different joint parts in contact with each other.

OSTEOPOROSIS: weakening of the bones related to a decrease in bone density.

PHYTOTHERAPY: medicine which treats or prevents diseases by using plants.

PHLEBITIS: formation of a blood clot inside a vein which harms circulation.

POLYPHENOLS: natural substances present in many plants (fruits, vegetables, herbs, cereals and grains) which have an antioxidant action.

FREE RADICALS: unstable molecules released by a reaction involving oxygen in the body (for example, production of energy) which can damage cells by trying to stabilize themselves.

RHEUMATISM: terms which includes all of the acute or chronic diseases which affect the joints.

MOTHER TINCTURE: medical preparation obtained by dissolving the active ingredients of a plant or a mineral after maceration in alcohol.

TRIGLYCERIDES: molecules which store and transport fats in the body.

ULCER: loss of the mucous membrane which covers the body (skin) or internal parts of the body (intestine or stomach).

VITAMIN: molecule indispensable for functioning of the body which it cannot synthesize. It must contributed by the diet.

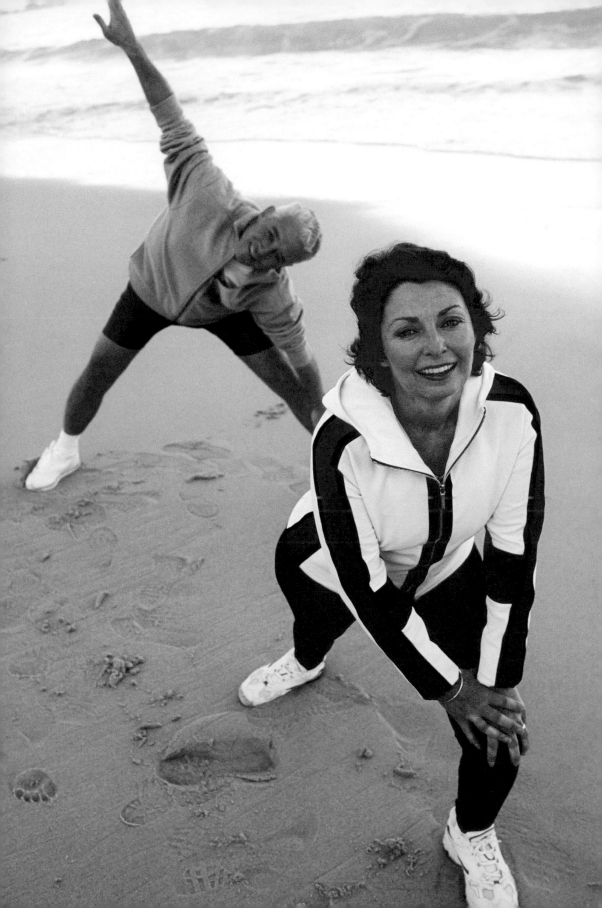

BIBLIOGRAPHY

Publications

Allemand H., Roussille B.: *Mal de dos: ouvrons le dialogue.* Comité Français d'Éducation de la Santé. Paris, 2002.

Borel M.: *Ces plantes qui nous veulent du bien.* Albin Michel, Paris, 1998.

Botticelli A.M.: *Les Plantes médicinales.* Gründ, Paris, 1999.

Dufour A., Festy D.: *Toujours jeune grâce aux compléments alimentaires.* Marabout, Paris, 2003.

Gerber N.: *Livre de poche de rhumatologie.* Flammarion, Paris, 1995.

Hazeltine M.: *Guide pratique de rhumatologie.* Gaëtan Morin, Paris, 1990.

Massol M.: *La Nutrimédecine.* PUF, Paris, 1998.

Pallardy P.: *Plus jamais mal au dos.* Laffont, Paris, 2000.

Perrot S.: *Med-Line de rhumatologie.* Estem, Paris, 1996.

Théodosaki J.: *L'Arthrose.* Édition de Falbis, Paris, 1998.

Studies

Berenbaum F.: *Anti-inflammatoires.* La revue du Praticien 1er mars 2003, tome 53, n° 6: 703-707.

Blankenhorn G.: *Clinical effectiveness of Spondyvit (vitamin E) in activated arthroses. A multicenter placebo-controlled double-blind study.* Z Ort hop 1986, 124 (3): 340-343.

Burrows M.: *Physiological factors associated with low bone mineral density in female endurance runners.* Br J Sports Med 2003, 37 (1): 67-71.

Chantre P.: *Efficacy and tolerance of Harpagophytum procumbens versus diacerhein in treatment of osteoarthritis.* Phytomedicine 2000, 7(3): 177-183.

Chevalier: *Arthrose.* La Revue du Praticien 15 mars 2003, tome 53, n° 6: 512- 515.

Criswell L.A.: *Cigarette smoking and the risk of rheumatoid arthritis among postmenopausal women: results from the Iowa Women's Health Study.* Am J Med 2002, 112(6): 465-71.

Curtis C.: *The effect of Omega-3 polyunsaturated fatty acids on degenerative joint disease.* Agrofood industry hi tech 2003: 22-25.

Ettinger W.H. Jr : *A randomized trial comparing aerobic exercise and resistance exercise with a health education program in older adults with knee osteoarthritis.* The Fitness Arthritis and Seniors Trial (FAST). JAMA 1997, 277(1) : 25-31.

Hurley M.V. : *Improvements in quadriceps sensorimotor function and disability of patients with knee osteoarthritis following a clinically practicable exercise regime.* Br J Rheumatol. 1998, 37(11) : 1181-1187.

Jensen N.H. : *Reduced pain from osteoarthritis in hip joint or knee joint during treatment with calcium ascorbate. A randomized, placebo-controlled cross-over trial in general practice* Ugeskr Laeger. 2003, 165(25) : 2563-2566.

Long L. : *Herbal medicines for the treatment of osteoarthritis: a systematic review.* Rheumatology 2001, 40: 779-793.

Machtey I. : *Tocopherol in Osteoarthritis: a controlled pilot study.* J Am Geriatr Soc 1978, 26(7) : 328-330.

McAlindon T.E. : *Do antioxidant micronutrients protect against the development and progression of knee osteoarthritis ?* Arthritis Rheum 1996, 39(4) : 648-656.

Mc Alindon T. : *Glucosamine and chondroitin for treatment of osteoarthritis.* JAMA 2000, 283(11) : 1-12.

Reginster J.Y. : *The prevalence and burden of arthritis.* Rheumatology (Oxford) 2002, 41 Suppl 1 : 3-6.

Reginster J.-Y. : *Les Propriétés de la glucosamine.* J. Pharm Belg 2000, 55(5) : 118-121.

Scherak O. : *High dosage vitamin E therapy in patients with activated arthrosis.* Z Rheumatol 1990, 49 (6): 369-373.

Shepard G. : *Ex-professional association footballers have an increased prevalence of osteoarthritis of the hip compared with age matched controls despite not having sustained notable hip injuries.* Br J Sports Med 2003, 37(1) : 80-81.

Vincent K.R. : *Resistance exercise and bone turnover in elderly men and women.* Med Sci Sports Exerc 2002, 34(1) : 17-23.

From Inuit to implementation: omega-3 fatty acids come of age. Mayo Clin Proc. 2000, 75 (6): 607-614.

Henrotin, Y. : *Avocado/soybean unsaponifiables prevent the inhibitory effect of osteoarthritic subchondral osteoblasts on aggrecan and type II collagen synthesis by chondrocytes.* J Rheumatol, 2006. In Press

Useful websites

- www.apta.org

- www.arthrolink.com

- www.aapmr.org

- www.capmr.ca

In our collection Alpen éditions:

-Osteoarthrisis, Rheumatism, Arthritis

-Osteoporosis

-Control your acidity, the acid/base diet

-Handle your menopause

-The Omega-3 Answer

-Living with a Hyperactive Child

-All About the Prostate

-The French Paradox

-The XXL Syndrome

with Michel Montignac:

-The French GI Diet for Women

-Eat Yourself Slim

-The Montignac Diet Cookbook

-The French GI Diet

-Glycemic Index Diet

www.alpen.mc